Real Life Diaries

THROUGH THE EYES
OF DID

True stories about dissociative identity disorder and living with multiple parts, alters, identities & personalities

LYNDA CHELDELIN FELL

with

SUNSHINE PURCELL

AMELIA JOUBERT

COVER ART BY ANDRE
Denise Purcell's alter

TRIGGER WARNING
This book contains potentially distressing content to readers who live with dissociative identity disorder.
READ WITH CAUTION

A portion of proceeds from the sale of this book is donated to National Alliance for Mental Illness, a not-for-profit organization dedicated to building better lives for the millions affected by mental illness. For more information, visit www.nami.org.

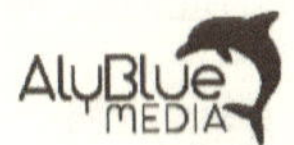

Real Life Diaries
Through the Eyes of DID – 1st ed.
True stories about dissociative identity disorder and living with multiple parts, alters, identities & personalities
Lynda Cheldelin Fell/Sunshine Purcell/Amelia Joubert
Real Life Diaries www.RealLifeDiaries.com

Cover Design by AlyBlue Media, LLC
Interior Design by AlyBlue Media LLC
Published by AlyBlue Media, LLC

ISBN: 978-1-944328-83-2
Library of Congress Control Number: 2016919552
AlyBlue Media, LLC
Ferndale, WA 98248
www.AlyBlueMedia.com

This book is designed to provide informative narrations to readers. It is sold with the understanding that the writers, authors or publisher is not engaged to render any type of psychological, legal, or any other kind of professional advice. The content is the sole expression and opinion of the authors and writers. No warranties or guarantees are expressed or implied by the choice to include any of the content in this book. Neither the publisher nor the author or writers shall be liable for any physical, psychological, emotional, financial, or commercial damages including but not limited to special, incidental, consequential or other damages. Our views and rights are the same: You are responsible for your own choices, actions and results.

PRINTED IN THE UNITED STATES OF AMERICA

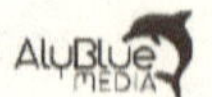

ii

Through the Eyes of DID

DEDICATION

This book is dedicated to all who
live with dissociative identity disorder

THROUGH THE EYES OF DID

Through the Eyes of DID

CONTENTS

BY LYNDA CHELDELIN FELL

PREFACE

In 1973, when the book *Sybil* was released, the world was captivated. Written by Flora Rheta Schreiber, it featured a patient diagnosed with dissociative identity disorder, known back then as multiple personalities. The story was so strange and unique that it was made into a television movie in 1976, and again in 2007. The good news is that *Sybil* opened the dialogue on a little understood mental illness. The bad news is that decades later, the portrayal remains the same: misunderstood and sometimes villainized.

Fast forward to 2015. I first met Sunshine when she registered under the name Denise Purcell to share her story about losing a daughter in Grief Diaries. Although her story was sad, I was struck by her writing. Between the lines I found a lovely, compassionate soul. We bonded immediately. Months later, Sunshine bravely shared with me that there are multiple alters—seventeen parts—who reside within Denise. I discovered that I had never actually met Denise, and all my interactions had been with her host alter, Sunshine. I knew her condition stemmed from childhood trauma, but that was all I knew and I left it at that. To me, Sunshine hadn't changed since revealing her condition. She was still Sunshine, and I adored her.

I've since met a few more alters, each of whom is unique and special in his and her own way. Collectively, they comprise a wise and compassionate friend whom I've come to admire and love.

It's been decades since *Sybil* was released, and yet those who live with DID continue to face deep societal stigma. They're often accused of being crazy, feared, or just downright fake. I hope this book changes that. The writers have faced tremendous challenges throughout life with little support, yet each courageously bares all in this book with hopes of helping others like them feel less alone, and for the rest of us to better understand.

Skeptics can be masterful spinners, so a few things are worth noting. First, when a writer contradicts themselves, it's not because they're lying. It's because a different alter is answering, and he or she has a different perspective. Second, the analogy of a car or bus is used by multiple writers to describe what it's like to live with DID. This analogy is used repeatedly because it works.

The writers understand that bravely sharing their private stories puts them at risk for more judgment, and yet they share anyway to help make a difference. They are true pioneering heroes.

Although most who live with DID suffered severe childhood trauma, this book isn't about the trauma. Our purpose is to fight stigma, open the door to compassion by raising awareness, and offer comfort to others who share their path.

Welcome to our village.

Warm regards,

Lynda Cheldelin Fell
Creator, Grief Diaries

BY SUNSHINE PURCELL

INTRODUCTION

I became acquainted with Lynda Cheldelin Fell while contributing to the book *Grief Diaries: Surviving Loss of a Child*. Through emails we developed a close friendship. I found that Lynda believed in helping others through sharing stories and experiences. This book, *Through the Eyes of DID,* also known as dissociative identity disorder, is a compilation of personal stories written by those who live with DID. This book is about how people with this disorder live, struggle, and survive each day in a world that seems to know so little about the subject. This is a real, painful truth we live with each day. As children, our minds could not cope with the traumatic circumstances, not being able to comprehend the abuse, so our minds created a safe haven and split off into a personality to deal with such horrendous circumstances. This is a coping mechanism.

As we get older and trauma is still occurring in our lives, we create more personalities to deal with it. Some of our personalities are developed just to function in the world and do daily tasks. Some personalities are fragmented and have no perception of the consequences of their own actions. Some are developed to get through social functions, family gatherings and such, and don't hold a trauma at all. This is a way of life.

There are symptoms of eating disorders, relationship issues, gender issues, severe depression, posttraumatic stress disorder and pseudo seizures that come about through emotional stress and suppressing the trauma we endured. There is a significant amount of therapy needed along with medication, but every case is an individual one and should be treated as such. There is no cure. It may be manageable if all personalities are on board and living co-consciously with the others, but that can take years or even a lifetime. It's learning to live in a world that knows very little about the disorder. Many people are misinformed, and we are often misdiagnosed. But one thing is certain: most of us who live with DID are unique and talented.

My greatest hope is that you will read this book and have better understanding and compassion when it comes to people living with this disorder. You can have a meaningful life both living with this or having a relationship with us.

My name is Sunshine, my birth name is Denise. I have dissociative identity disorder. We are seventeen personalities living in one body. There is sadness and a lot of love in this book. I thank everyone who participated, because I know how hard it is to keep focused most of the time. I thank Lynda for having the compassion and courage to help us tell each of our stories. I thank her for giving me the gift of friendship. That is a true blessing when you have lived a sheltered life. Lynda means the world to me.

I hope you enjoy this compilation of stories about us. "Strength comes in numbers; we are many." If you would like to learn more about my life, join us on Sister Diaries with Sunshine on YouTube.

Much love,

SUNSHINE
Denise Purcell's host alter

THROUGH THE EYES OF DID

GLOSSARY

ALTERS: Alters are dissociated parts of the self who operate and perceive the world independent of one another. Alters have different names, genders, ages, birthdates, skills, memories, triggers, and responsibilities. Some alters are more communicative. Some rarely, if ever, front. Alters can be related. For example, two of Denise Purcell's young alters, five-year-old Sarah and seven-year-old Abbey, are sisters. When Sarah fronts, Abbey is always close behind.

CO-CONSCIOUS: Otherwise known as co-con, this refers to the ability of two or more alters to be aware of the outside world at the same time.

CORE: The core is the original part of the self that existed before the alters came into being. A core is different from the host. Depending on the system, the core may retreat so deeply that they rarely or never front.

DISSOCIATING: Dissociation is a mental process that allows a person to disconnect from thoughts, emotions, memories, and actions as a way to mentally escape fear and pain during trauma. Most individuals who develop DID have a history of repetitive, overwhelming, and often life-threatening trauma at a young age.

DOUBLE SWITCH: The ability to switch between alters very fast and undetected.

FLASHBACKS: Flashbacks occur when a dissociated memory rises to the surface, involuntarily transporting the alter back in time. The alter is forced to relieve the intense event as if it were actually occurring.

FRAGMENT: A fragment is an alter who is not fully developed, physically and/or consciously. Fragments may exist to carry out a single function, or to hold a single memory or emotion. For example, one of Denise Purcell's alters has only an upper body, yet he serves a role within her system.

FRONTING: Alters who "front" take control of the body and the conscious part of the mind.

HOST: The host is the alter who is in control of the body and is conscious more than other alters. The host alter is often responsible for activities of daily living, though some of this may be supported by other alters. The host may or may not be the individual's original personality.

INSIDE FAMILIES: See "system."

INTEGRATE: Integration is when an alter absorbs into the individual, becoming a part and no longer a separate personality or identity.

INTROJECT: An internal projected image. Introjects are alters who were split off to represent outside people, most typically an abuser

LITTLES: Alters who are young.

MULTIPLE: DID was known as multiple personality disorder until 1994. "Multiple" is shorthand for someone with dissociative identity disorder.

OTHERS: Same as "alters."

PARTS: Same as "alters."

PLEURAL: Term used by people with DID to describe themselves.

POLYFRAGMENTED: Generally accepted definition for those with over 100 alters.

SINGLETON: Term used by people with DID to describe those who don't live with DID.

SWITCHING: Switching refers to one alter taking or gaining control of the body. Switches can be consensual, forced, or triggered. If two alters choose to switch with each other, they usually have some degree of co-consciousness with each other. The alter who steps back might no longer be aware of the outside world.

SUBSYSTEMS: Subsystems are separate internal groups within one system. Groups from different subsystems may not be aware of one another. Groups may have good communication and co-consciousness among themselves, but may lose time when alters from other subsystems front. Subsystems may reside in different locations in an internal world, or may have non-overlapping internal worlds. Some subsystems might be entirely trauma-locked; for example, someone with DID might have a group of alters who experience themselves as permanently trapped in an abusive environment, can only rarely communicate with the main group of alters, and cannot understand that the body is no longer trapped and hurting.

SYSTEM: The system refers to all the alters together in one body, though not all who live with DID are aware of their system. Systems are also called collectives, internal or inside families, clans, or crews.

TRAUMA: A severely distressing experience resulting from acute physical or emotional pain that produces overwhelming feelings of terror, horror, or helplessness.

TRIGGERS: Trigger is a term referring to any stimulus that evokes a memory. Being aware of triggers allows an alter to prepare for it sometimes, but doesn't make it go away or lessen. For instance, if loud noises are a trigger, one might help cope with the Fourth of July by wearing earplugs.

In the Mind of a Child
BY SUNSHINE

In the mind of a child,
so innocent and free
always exciting new days
awaiting to see.

Sweet innocence that
nothing can compare
the world is a safe place,
as long as you are there.

Taking their hand,
so soft, so small,
right there to catch them
if they happen to fall.

The feeling oh I can do anything,
just let me try
with warm hugs and kisses
that can stop any cry.

No worries, no pain
that hold them back,
full of love and wonder,
there is nothing they lack.

The smell of their skin
so sweet and new,
and when you're feeling down
they are right beside you.

So give them a safe place
to have and to hold
and watch as they flourish,
and start to unfold.

In the mind of a child
so innocent and free
I once knew her,
that child was me.

CHAPTER ONE

The Beginning

The thing that is really hard, and really amazing, is giving up on being perfect and beginning the work of becoming yourself. -ANNA QUINDLEN

Formerly known as multiple personalities, dissociative identity disorder is a unique diagnosis in which one body is shared between two or more personalities. Often referred to as "alters," each one has its own disposition and persona. Some have full identities, some do not. Most have names and distinct ages, but not all. In this chapter, each writer shares the beginning of his or her journey through living with DID.

*

ADRIANNE ALLEN-LANG
Adrianne was diagnosed with 10
personalities in 2015 at age 18

My parents split when I was two and a half years old. The night before my mother left is my earliest memory, and is the night when I birthed my dissociative identity disorder. I remember walking out to speak with my parents and asking them to stop yelling, because I was trying to sleep. My mother put me back to bed, and when I woke up again she was gone.

For the next ten years I bounced between my parents who couldn't be within meters of each other. I have many memories of them screaming at one another outside the car during custody exchanges. It was so bad that my father would not come to any of my school award ceremonies, all because my mother would be there and he'd start a scene.

My father was never involved with us very much, and would buy us expensive things so we wouldn't bother him. He moved to the city with us when I was nine. Prior to that we would go back down to the country town and spend every second weekend with him and his friend. When I was four his friend started molesting me, and I was too scared to say anything. Kitty was birthed to deal with the trauma.

My father also groomed me from a young age to prepare to leave my mum. He would always drill into my head that she hated my brother and me, and that we needed to be with him to be safe.

When I was twelve I moved from living with my mother full-time to living with my father, his girlfriend and her three kids. At this time I was in grade six of primary school and was getting bullied savagely. I was suicidal and using my dissociation and alters to get through each day. At this stage there were four of us including Az (host), Pumpkin (core), Kitty and Adrian. My father's girlfriend at the time, M, and her kids would beat me. If I ever fought back to the kids, M would beat me even more and force me to do everyone's chores while her kids got to lounge around and throw things at me.

When I started high school (middle school for anyone outside of Australia) the bullying escalated and I was given the typical response, "What did you do to provoke them?"

"Just move away."

"That doesn't sound like the truth."

"Your fault for having your bra showing."

My first year of high school birthed my fifth alter, Anna, a mute that I used to survive the bullying. I was thrown off moving buses, had my things stolen and thrown in trees, as well as a barrage of verbal and physical abuse. The second year of high school birthed number six, named Keegan. He started a lot of problems including fighting, violence, drugs, and alcohol.

One afternoon during class, a child was hitting me in the back. After warning him three times to stop, we just snapped and belted the life out of him. We had to be pulled off by two other male students, and that was the end of that high school. After being removed from there I suffered a psychotic breakdown where I had to be sectioned (detained under the Mental Health Act) for a week due to being a threat to myself and apparently others. I was held down and had my piercings ripped out of my ears, and was handcuffed to a hospital bed and ambulance gurney, all because I wanted to be left alone.

My diary was found, telling about my self-harming, suicide and others in my head, but it was used against me instead of to help me, I was thirteen at this time. This started a downward spiral of impulsive, reckless relationships, underage prostitution, and drug abuse, which didn't ease up until my second pregnancy. During this stage I became pregnant with my first son due to a drug-hazed rape. I was belted within an inch of my life during school when I was seventeen weeks pregnant, and miscarried due to it. My alter Allie came about from this, the motherly feminist.

I went home to my father. His girlfriend pinned me up against a wall by my throat, told me I was a disgrace, useless, and to leave and never come back, or she would kill me. I went back to my mother for a bit but the local abuse escalated and I couldn't cope, so I fled across the country to where I met my son's father. He was highly physically, mentally, emotionally and financially abusive to me, as well as being a hardcore drug addict. I was too scared to leave, and at twelve weeks pregnant with my son, after a hospital stay and nearly losing him, I came home to abuse again. My son's father spent eight hundred dollars on drugs and then started on me. He punched a hole through a wall and left me screaming in a corner, crying out that I'd rather kill myself and our baby than spend another second with him.

Suddenly it was like I was in a haze as I left him. I hated what I was doing, but I couldn't stop, even as he was laying into me. I just kept moving around and packing up, protecting my stomach. I have since found out that it was an alter who ultimately saved my life and my child's. Without my head mates, I believe we'd be dead either at the hands of my son's father, or by our own. I have an introject (an internal projected image of an abuser) of my son's father; his name is Muscle. Muscle torments me with nightmares and traumatic flashbacks, which means I don't sleep much.

Since becoming a mother at sixteen, there have been more experiences of abuse that have not birthed new alters, but brought pre-existing ones to the surface. It is constantly a learning experience, especially when new rooms or things pop up in my inner world. There are currently ten of us including Az, Adrianne, Kitty, Pumpkin, Keegan, Muscle, Nurse, Harley, Myrnin and Anna, And I have no doubt you'll hear from them throughout this book.

*

GAIL BUSWELL
Gail was diagnosed with 13
personalities in 2002 at age 24

My DID story is a very painful and debilitating one, and I only know the tip of the iceberg. I have very little to no memory of my childhood. Hundreds of photos but no concrete memories. To the outside world my life was perfect. I lived with my mum, dad, and three siblings. We lived in a posh house and my dad was a very well known and loved bishop of my local church. I attended a private school and wanted for nothing. But the reality was that I was born into a cult led by my father (the title of father is now stripped from him). I suffered unspeakable satanic ritual abuse at the hands of my abusers.

In September 1999, my main abuser was arrested and sentenced to eighteen years in prison. He was tried on evidence alone and the verdict was unanimous. My world temporarily fell apart. My family disowned me, and I coped by spending the next two years traveling the world. I have little memory of that time but tons of pictures. Upon my return I moved away from my hometown, leaving my past behind.

Life was good. We kept to ourselves. I was unique but very successful in my job. I was married and had three children. We, my internal system, worked well as a team. We participated in numerous activities and had many hobbies.

Fast-forward to 2015. Our abuser was due for parole. My life as I knew it was over. I was contacted to inform me of his release. Alters who had lain dormant became scared and active. My life became a living hell. New evidence was found against my abuser, and incriminated six other men too. After three months of painful questioning and my being forced to remember snippets of hell, our main abuser and his band of merry men will be incarcerated for life. My life went from bad to worse. I became an inpatient ten months ago and have yet to go home. I lost my children and my husband. My diagnoses are dissociative identity disorder, complex post-traumatic stress disorder, and emotionally unstable personality disorder with comorbidity of depression and anxiety.

*

KATT HART
Katt was diagnosed with hundreds
of personalities in 2011 at age 20

I was badly abused from age two by my grandparents and some people they knew. They recognized what they were doing to me, that they were creating different alters within me. I don't know how many they made or why they kept doing this sort of thing. Eventually we moved a long way away from where they lived, which stopped them from hurting us.

My parents neglected me. They were always busy with other things, and I was looked after by relatives and family friends, many of whom were abusive. I was sexually abused and bullied by other children, as well. I was emotionally abused by my parents.

In my teen years I got into multiple abusive relationships, most of them sexually abusive, and some were most emotionally abusive. Some of them found out about my alters and used that against us. They had taken advantage of the fact that many of my alters were very sexual or terrified to say no.

When I was eighteen I started to figure out that I had DID. It was hard, and I was in denial a lot for a couple of years until I was diagnosed. I haven't been able to access any therapy, as most are too expensive or won't treat someone with DID. All the progress I've made has been made alone or with the help of the few understanding people I've met over the last few years.

In the recent past we haven't had anyone who is out the most, so we don't have a host or anyone who even identifies with the body that we're in, but we make the best out of what we have. We switch alters often, but we have supportive people who are helping alters break out of the bad things they were taught and the roles they were given. Now we have a wonderful partner who has helped us all so much and loves us all a lot. We're still healing and still recovering memories, which means we're still finding dormant alters all the time. There are at least a few hundred, I think, that are written down in our journals. It's hard to keep track, but we are doing the best we can with the few resources we have access to.

*

ROSEMARY HAWKINS
Rosemary was diagnosed with at
least 5 personalities in 2014 at age 46

My story into my DID diagnosis began quite recently, but its origins occurred when I was young. From age five to fourteen I was sexually assaulted by my father. When I was five, my younger brother was born, and that was the catalyst for all my problems. With an emotionally detached and often absent mother, and a father as my abuser, I grew up without the core sense of security and love that children need.

I became a mini-mother to my siblings. I cooked, cleaned up afterward, and became a protector to them. And I began a complicated relationship with myself. I married and started my own family as soon as I was seventeen, and escaped my childhood that way. Through three marriages and five children, I had little time or inclination to explore the frailties I knew I had in myself. I was completely disconnected.

In 2008 my husband was diagnosed with pancreatic cancer and given three to six months to live. This rocked my world to its very foundation. When he died ten months after his diagnosis, I died on the inside. In the years since, I've had four nervous breakdowns and spent time in psychiatric hospitals.

My diagnosis of DID came in 2014 after spending four years lost in a haze of confusion, self-doubt, self-harm, and an increasing pattern of lost hours, even days at a time, items in my possession that I didn't recognize or remember, and journal writings that didn't make sense to me.

I now know that as a small child I adapted to the abuse and lack of security around me by dissociating. In a way, I had always known that I used this as a coping mechanism, and on the surface I would say that it served me well over the years. Being able to disconnect when things get overwhelming can be an effective solution.

The blow came in 2014 when amid my grief, a frightened little five-year-old girl started writing in my journal. When I woke each morning, my journal would be filled with a childish handwriting that I didn't recognize. This child wrote that she was frightened and wanted me to help her. When I faced this little girl in therapy, my psychologist startled me with the idea that this little girl lived inside me.

In a very short space of time, just a couple of months, we identified five alters. The first is the little girl who doesn't have a name. Second is Bel, who strongly identifies with Satan and refuses to step inside a church. Third is Rose, the all-caring, all-competent mother who looks after everyone else except herself. Fourth and fifth are two distinct others, one who identifies as male and another whom I know very little about yet.

I have lived my life to date in a completely disconnected and disjointed way. The result is that I have missed out on many of my children's special moments. I was there physically, but dis-connected in my head. I feel like my life has simply been a series of disjointed scenes that lack cohesion and fluidity, and I feel like I have been robbed of my sense of self and my place in the world.

*

AMELIA JOUBERT
Amelia was diagnosed with 12
personalities in 2013 at age 15

Dissociative identity disorder is caused by childhood trauma. I went through sexual trauma as a child, resulting in DID. It's a way to survive when a child has no way of escaping traumatic situations. My mind found a rather creative way to escape the trauma but because of this amazing survival technique, I didn't remember most of my trauma until a few years ago. Having dissociative identity disorder makes things more complicated sometimes, but it also saved my life.

I was fifteen when I was diagnosed with DID and it was hard to accept, but also a huge relief to know what was going on with me. After years of hearing people talking in my head, having days I couldn't remember and having people tell me I did things I had no memory of doing, I finally had an answer.

There are twelve main identities, or alters, including myself. All the identities as a whole are referred to as a system. Tina is the youngest at four years old. She is very sweet and has a Southern accent. As far as we know, she doesn't hold much trauma but she does hold some emotional trauma. She loves horses and kittens.

Next is Snake, age five. His job is to cheer up the sad people in our system. He is a very happy little boy and he loves to make others happy. He loves reptiles, dragons, and science.

K is six. She is a very happy and fun-loving kid who sees good in the world and doesn't hold bad memories of any kind. She loves to play, eat sweets, and baby animals. She loves fairies.

Blossom is fourteen. She is sweet and shy. Her job in the system is to take care of the children. She is very nurturing and always looks out for the kids' best interests.

Rider, also fourteen, is a typical teenage boy. He likes to skateboard and is dating another alter in my system, named May. She is sixteen and rebellious, but tries to keep out of trouble for the sake of our system. She isn't a fan of drama and likes to just have fun.

Next is Ahina, age eighteen. She is the twin sister of Jax. She has a Southern accent. Ahina is our verbal protector and she will stand up to anyone who is verbally being mean or aggressive toward us. She likes things a certain way and likes to clean.

Jax, also eighteen, is our physical protector. If we feel threatened physically he will come out to protect us. He is quiet and keeps to himself. He is a great artist and loves to draw. He also loves music, especially rock.

Then there is me, Amelia. I am eighteen and I enjoy reading and writing. I also love animals.

Next is Scarlet, age nineteen. She is very outgoing and energetic. She loves meeting new people and being the life of the party. She shares my passion for educating people on mental health conditions.

Last is John, age twenty-four. He is like a big brother figure to our system and has a strong moral compass that helps keep us all on the straight and narrow. John is gay and is a big LGBT+ activist. He likes to cook and do hair.

We are a family, and all look out for one another.

*

AMANDA LINEBACK
Amanda was diagnosed with hundreds
of personalities in 2013 at age 31

I was born October 15,1982, at 7:04 p.m. I was premature and spent my first days of life in an incubator. I experienced my first trauma in my first few weeks of life. My incubator malfunctioned, causing the temperature to rise. I lay there helpless, being cooked alive, as nurses passed me by unaware of what was happening. My father saved my life that day when he came to look at me through the nursery window. He noticed that my body was red as a lobster and I looked limp and lifeless. He slammed his fists on the nursery window until he got the attention of a nurse, who saved me from certain demise. I think that my dad was showing genuine love for me that day, but looking back, it would have been less cruel for him to let me die. I was a victim of cult-oriented ritual satanic abuse, programming, and mind control until I was five years old, when my father went to prison for murder.

My first memory of being abused is when I was around four years old. I was taking a bath and my father came in and made me touch myself. He forced himself into my mouth, and I passed out because I couldn't breathe. He told me I was his special little girl and that I can't tell anyone because he wanted me to himself. He got me out of the tub and said I couldn't look pretty because then someone else might want to touch me. He made me cut my hair so short that I looked like a little boy. I got dressed, and he took me to get ice cream as a reward.

I am not sure how old I was when the rituals started, but I was very small. There were tables lined up that had straps and chains that were used to position you in various ways. There were many adults, but I could only see their eyes because they wore masks. When you were strapped onto the table you got blindfolded. I remember hearing other children crying and screaming in pain. I knew better than to make a sound. If you couldn't dissociate, you were on the list to be sacrificed. There were times when I was covered in blood from head to toe and forced to participate in the torture of other children. The adults would sometimes have knives on their fingers and privates. There was a different type of sexual, spiritual, and physical abuse for every occasion.

My mother had to work so much to make ends meet that we sometimes had two or three babysitters a day. The time between my dad going to prison and my mother meeting my soon-to-be stepdad was the happiest time of my childhood. My mommy was a rock star. She cuddled with us every night, gave us kisses and hugs whenever we wanted, and made me feel safe and loved. She protected us like she was a lioness and we were her cubs.

My mom and stepdad got married when I was close to seven years old. From the time they got married until I was eighteen, my life was a chaotic whirlwind of neglect, abandonment, and physical, emotional, verbal, and sexual abuse. I was forced to grow up too early, pushed away, treated as if I was unlovable, not good enough, and no one cared if my life amounted to anything. I was molested by so many caregivers that I don't know how many times it happened. I was mistreated to the point where I began to believe I deserved to be treated like an object. I lost the ability to love myself. Each time I was abused, a piece of my spirit was taken from me until the only thing left was an empty shell. I felt broken on the inside and lost on the outside. If someone had told me that I was abused as a child, I would have called him or her a liar. I thought I had a pretty normal life, with the exception of a few incidents. I went to college, fell in love, got married, and had my daughter and son. In 2011, I went through a very painful divorce and was alienated by my entire family. In the search for a new place to live I met my hero, Chad Funke.

Chad and I went on our first date on May 26, 2011, and I knew he was going to be my hero. Chad is the reason I am here today. He has been with me every step of this journey and has saved my life in more than one way.

I had no idea that I had a trauma volcano brewing inside of me and when it erupted, it did not hold back. The night it happened, Chad was working on one of his houses about twenty miles away. I don't remember driving to where he was, and I don't remember what happened before I drove to see him. I showed up and started frantically beating on the door. Chad opened the door and looked at me in disbelief, because I was standing there with a bloody knife in my hand, begging him to take it from me. I had cut myself two hundred and fifty times from the knee to the upper thigh on each leg. My shoulders, chest, stomach, arms, legs, and feet were covered with more cuts than I had visible skin.

That was the day my mental well-being became the focus of Chad's life. He called every mental health provider in my area to get me an appointment. I lost days at a time and had no control over what I was doing because I kept reliving flashbacks. I finally was safe enough that my body decided it was time to heal. The horrors of my childhood were playing out each day right in front of me. Chad stayed with me and took care of me day and night without ever making me feel bad or guilty. He made sure my children were taken care of, and protected them from being exposed to anything traumatic. It took four months for me to get into a therapist, and Chad never left my side. He is the other part of my heart and the absolute light in my life. He is my best friend, and I can never thank him enough for what he has done for me. It took nearly two years of flashbacks, nightmares, panic attacks, therapy appointments, and medication failures before I was sitting in Dr. Gable's office the day I received my diagnosis.

*

JANE MACDONALD
Jane was diagnosed with 3 personalities in
2014 at age 35, and currently has 6 alters

The story of my journey with DID is a lot less clear-cut and straightforward than some of the other ones in this book. Although abuse did happen—I am not a fan of using that word to describe what happened to me—a large part of my history is a blank. Some of the parts I do remember are fuzzy, and some events blur together. I know that this is a coping mechanism and is part of my mind's way of dealing with the traumas that occurred, just as developing other personalities is another way of dealing with the abuse that happened. I can't tell you stories of horrendous abuse that clearly explain why I am the way that I am. All I can offer you are the bits and pieces that I have remembered.

I grew up in a broken home. My parents separated when I was five, and I have no recollection of what life was like with them together. Their divorce was finalized when I was around eight or nine.

I lived with my emotionally abusive mother and my twin sister. We spent one evening each week visiting my dad at his house, as well as alternating weekends and holidays.

It was not a happy childhood. My mother verbally and emotionally attacked me on a regular basis, and my father engaged in certain inappropriate sexual acts with me starting around age six or so. I have a hard time using the word "abuse" to describe the behavior of either of my parents, because I have read and heard of parents who have done things far worse. I feel that even though my parents' behavior may now be labeled as abuse, I never thought of it as such. I didn't think it was normal; I just thought it was part of life, something you learn to live with, something you endure.

Around the same time my father began to do inappropriate things, I was also being abused by the son of a family friend. To start, the abuse took the form of verbal and emotional attacks. He said I was ugly, useless, fat, stupid, and worthless. He told me how embarrassing it was to be seen with me, and that he tolerated my presence only because my parents were friends of his parents. I hated being forced to see him, but because my parents were such close friends with his and had no idea what he was doing and saying to me. I was forced to visit him almost every week.

Frankly, I was too ashamed to say anything. I also bought into what he was saying to me, because I was also being bullied and given the same messages from my schoolmates and my mother. I begged my mom not to make me go with her when she visited his parents, but my requests fell on deaf ears. The teasing and insults only got worse over time. And then things took an even worse turn. He started touching me and forcing me to touch him in a sexual way. I told him I didn't want to, but I had no choice. He threatened me. I was too scared and ashamed to say anything, so it went on for years until I was a teenager and he lost interest in me.

Although my DID diagnosis is fairly recent, I noticed signs of it throughout my youth and into adulthood, but never knew what they meant. I found myself waking up in places, and not remembering how I got there or how long I had been there. I remember feeling like a completely different person in certain places and at certain times, transforming from a painfully shy and introverted individual to a highly talkative and social person. I noticed things in my belongings that I did not purchase and had not received as gifts. I even had people claim to know me but whom I did not recognize. Inexplicably, these people would know things about me such as where I lived, where I went to school, and more, yet I had no recollection of who they were or ever having met them before. Other times I simply felt not real, as if I was in somebody else's body. I also began noticing periods of lost time, sometimes a few minutes and sometimes several hours. For these periods of time I would simply have no memory of what I had done or said, or where I had been.

I had never heard about dissociative identity disorder, or multiple personality disorder as it was once called, and so I never knew what all these things meant. They were just the way it was. After studying psychology I was aware of the existence of DID, but I never thought to apply that label to myself. We were always warned about the dangers of self-diagnosing, and I always thought of it as something that happens to other people, not to me. However after being diagnosed with dissociative identity disorder, I can easily see that these experiences were really times when my other personalities took over and I would dissociate. Hindsight is always 20/20, though. Although I am not thrilled to have this diagnosis, I am learning to live with it.

At the time of my initial diagnosis, I knew of three alters: Clara, Angela, and Jack. Over time I have developed more alters and other alters seem to have merged together. At this point in my life it is myself (Jane), Clara, Emily, Jess, Angela, and Kali.

*

CRYSTALIE MATULEWICZ
Crystalie was diagnosed with dissociative
identity disorder in 2015 at age 29

To the outside world, it appeared as if I was growing up in a normal, loving family: a mother and father with two well-behaved children who attended private school, a family who attended church every Sunday and took part in community activities. But that was just a façade to cover up what was really going on behind closed doors: physical, sexual, and emotional abuse and neglect that continued for twenty-nine years resulting in my DID.

My biological mother was my main abuser. I call her my biological mother because it's difficult to call her my mother. I acknowledge that she gave birth to me, but her motherly qualities stopped there. For simplicity, I will refer to her as my mother, but I'd like to believe that real mothers don't abuse their children.

Growing up, I was not allowed to talk to outsiders. My mother told us that whatever happens in the family stays in the family. She convinced me that the world was a scary place, and that no one would understand me. I spent my childhood living in fear of my home and fear of the outside world. There was no safe space to exist. The way I survived was by splitting off into different parts. I would never have been able to handle all the trauma on my own.

I often refer to my home as a prison. It may not have been an eight-foot cell, but it was a prison; it just happened to have decent furniture. As a child, I felt trapped. There was no place to hide; even the closets were blocked off. Every night my mother slept just a few feet away from the front door, a practice she continued until the day I escaped. I could never run away. The only place I could escape to was inside my mind.

My older brother was the golden child. Although he was also abused, it was different; my mother disguised it as love. With me, there was no love. I was the evil child, the cause of all our family's problems. No matter what I did, I was wrong. If I didn't perform well, I wasn't good enough. If I did perform well, I was punished for thinking I was better than her. I was put in a lose-lose situation. As an adult, I learned that my mother was, and still is, a sociopath. As much as she made me believe the abuse was my fault, it never was. It was all part of her game.

As a child, I was never allowed to bathe alone. My mother was always there, sitting and watching me. She helped because she said I didn't know how to clean myself. I realized later on that it was her covert way of sexually abusing me. I was finally allowed to shower by myself when I became a teenager, but the damage was already done. To this day I still have flashbacks when I'm in the shower.

I also woke to my mother sexually abusing me. She told me I was sick and that she was trying to help. But I wasn't sick at all, and she was hurting me. Despite my pleas, she wouldn't stop. I'd go off to another place in my mind so I didn't have to focus on what was happening to me. I did this a lot during my childhood. At the time, I didn't know it had a name: dissociation.

I also experienced psychological abuse at the hands of my mother. She gave me toys only to destroy them right in front of me, telling me I didn't deserve them. One of my parts holds a memory of holding a ball while our mother stabbed it with a kitchen knife. If someone gave me a gift, my mother either destroyed it or took it for herself. She said I never deserved good things.

If my mother thought I was bad, she wouldn't allow me to eat. Sometimes it was just for a day, sometimes longer. When I could eat, she would give me food she knew I couldn't eat. I coped with feeling hungry by dissociating. Several of my parts and I still struggle with disordered eating because we have internalized our mother's belief that we are undeserving of food.

I experienced consistent physical abuse. I was rarely bad. I was a straight-A student, polite and kind-hearted, but that didn't matter. My mother always found something to punish me for, even if it was just something she made up to justify her actions. I was made to feel as if my existence was enough of a reason to be hurt.

My father was physically abusive as well, especially as I got older. The worst experience occurred when I was a teenager. My high school called my parents with a concern that I was depressed. I knew it was going to end up getting me in trouble. I went home from school that day in tremendous fear. I knew that look in my father's eyes; it was not a look of concern. It was a look of anger, the only emotion I ever saw in either of my parents.

I sat in the chair that night while my father beat me. I begged him to stop, and apologized for feeling depressed and offending the family. But my words didn't matter. My father told me he was going to give me something to be depressed about. He beat me but for how long, I do not know; there are still a lot of pieces I don't remember clearly. I know I started crying, and went completely numb. I felt nothing at all. No pain. No emotion. Nothing. I went through the next few years of my life shutting myself off from emotion, because feelings became a punishable offense.

Shortly after that experience I began hearing distinct voices. I didn't know what was going on at the time. I didn't want people to think I was crazy, so I never told anyone about the voice inside my head. He wasn't a bad voice. He was angry, just like me. Charlie became a welcome distraction from the horrors of my home life, which unfortunately didn't stop once I turned eighteen.

I continued to be physically, sexually, and emotionally abused into my adulthood, which is something I have had a hard time admitting. I was chronically ill throughout my adolescence and early twenties, which my mother used as an excuse to continually abuse me. It was so normalized that no one in my family even batted an eye. I kept forming parts to handle the continuing trauma, though I was still unaware of everything that was happening, both inside my mind and outside my body. I felt as if I was just stumbling through my life in a haze. It wasn't until my mid-twenties that I started remembering some of the childhood abuse; before then, my childhood memories were nonexistent. I noticed the voices in my head becoming more active. I started having flashbacks and experiencing body memories. I was in and out of therapy, received over a dozen different diagnoses, and was put on countless medications. Nothing helped. I was still hearing the voices, and I was still spacing out. I was also still being abused, which made my symptoms worse.

I ended up in and out of psychiatric hospitals in 2014 and 2015. I knew I couldn't continue living like that any longer. I needed help, but I could get it only if I could get away from my family. I packed two bags with clothes and shoes, and I snuck out of the prison I was forced to call home for twenty-nine years. I ran away from my abusive family, never to see them again. I thought I would be okay once I was free from the abuse. I didn't realize it at the time, but running away from home put my entire system into chaos. It was a huge change from what we were used to. Parts were confused and scared. I was losing time, and my emotions were all over the place. I struggled with suicidal thoughts which were confusing because I had just found freedom—the last thing I wanted to do was lose that. I didn't really understand what was going on until my therapist diagnosed me with DID. It has since been a journey of denial, understanding, acceptance, and recovery.

There is a still a lot of my childhood that I don't remember. There is still a large part of my system that I don't connect with. I don't talk about how many parts I have, because there are more than I'd like to admit. Not all have names, but each has a purpose. They all helped us survive.

*

ALICIA PETTIS
Alicia was diagnosed with 40
personalities in 2015 at age 16

When I was about age three my father began to abuse me. I grew up in a home that wasn't safe for my family. My father began abusing me when my mom took more work time to avoid being abused. His abuse started off happening only rarely, and then it flipped and occurred every night. It was physical, mental, and emotional. My first alter appeared when I was four after a year of daily abuse. Two years later I witnessed my father killing my baby brother and he blamed the death on the little six-year-old me. That's when my first child alter appeared. A few months later, after he was released, a third alter appeared. I wasn't conscious around that time. Having seen my brother's death forced me into hiding, and my child alter took over for me while I processed what I had seen.

Two-thirds of my abuse was split between my controlling father and my neglecting mother. The last third of my abuse came from outside sources that were either my father's doing or my mother's. From a very young age I learned that you can't trust many people, not even family, because they might hurt you. I learned to keep my mouth shut or else I'd be hurting, to stay in the shadows because too much spotlight might burn me. I was a child learning simple math and how to cover up marks.

*

SUNSHINE PURCELL
Denise was diagnosed with 17
personalities in 1995 at age 30

I was aware that I heard voices in my head, like statements that would respond to something I did. Or it would be the complete opposite of what I was thinking or doing. It didn't fit. I was told at times that I had a monotone voice and would react to things within seconds in a whole different manner. I have large amounts of time I can't account for during times of my childhood and adulthood. I have found myself in strange places, not knowing how I had arrived there. There are different styles of writings, music, foods, clothing styles, and talents. I wasn't aware why I had them.

I suffered from depression and hated being called by my birth name, Denise. There were times when I cried like a small child, or moaned in pain. I thought I was suffering from postpartum depression, so I sought therapy. After going through my childhood and revealing information I wasn't aware of, including a lot of abuse and dysfunction while growing up, I was diagnosed with DID. My grandfather molested me when I was a young child, and I have memories that date back to preverbal times. I can talk only about myself though, although more children in the family were involved.

I was diagnosed with dissociative identity disorder, post-traumatic stress disorder, and complex and severe depression. I have been in therapy for over twenty years and still have only scratched the surface. I have personalities that are female, male, children, Native American, a sailor with an Irish brogue, a sister and brother. They all serve a purpose, and that purpose was and still is to keep me alive.

I am not violent or bitter, and have been able to break the cycle of violence. I raised five girls who are independent and flourishing in their lives. But I deal with my DID every day. I didn't cause this, but I have to figure out how to maintain my life. That comes with struggles of not being able to have friends or be around people.

I question everything I do and feel, because what I feel isn't always my own. My parts all have their own personalities; they know each other and communicate, though not with me. I lose gaps of time and haven't been able to hold down a job since being diagnosed. They are part of me, and I wouldn't know how to live without them, nor would I want to. Because I have dissociative identity disorder and have been through the mental health system, I believe it's time for people to understand it's real and needs to be understood

*

ERICKA REEVE
Ericka was diagnosed with over
25 personalities in 2013 at age 26

One word comes to mind for me: inconsistency. I have lived through many things that I'm now more aware of due to years of therapy. I grew up on the south side of Chicago in a seemingly normal conservative Christian home. We were anything but your typical family, but from all appearances everything was kitties and rainbows.

Well, actually, not so much. Some days were good, even normal. But then the shift would happen. We'd go visit a grandmother, who is a sociopath and tortured us mercilessly. Yes, she is a sociopath. Torturing, tormenting and abandoning my mother and her siblings in ways you could likely never imagine possible. Now let that sink in a moment. This grandmother is one I was left with because, and I quote, "I wanted you to make your own decisions about her. I didn't want to get in the way of your relationship with her, and I thought you'd be okay because you were her granddaughter."

Pardon me, what? Many in my family are uneducated, and so it would seem that denial, and very clearly fear, are strong factors within the dynamic. I firmly believe that part of the reason I am a logical thinker is because of the brain I was born with, but also that I refused to be uninformed even at a very, very young age. My father's family were readers, and so I read anything I could. Everything. I read medical books, astrology books, psychology, sociology, novels, foreign literature, and so on. I read all of these things that held knowledge I could use, as well as my favorite book ever created: the dictionary.

Webster's Dictionary was always at my side. I read those books with Webster's right next to me. From some of these things and observations, one of my youngest and most intelligent parts was born. She is very young but in the few memories I have of her, I remember she was charming and pleasant and loved seeing her "little grandma's girl." But then my mother left, the doors closed (sometimes) and we would play one of her many games. That is where one of my more challenging parts came from. She is very much a mirror of my mother's mother. I use the terms mother, parent, grandmother and family very loosely, as you'll come to find. Family means nothing to me and my parts, because family is just something people say; words mean very little, actions count for something, not words.

As a result of weathering neglect from birth and severe abuse at the hands of multiple abusers through early childhood, both by family and not, I had no hope. It's as though the people in my life were trying to create a sociopath. I was treated like an animal by certain people. I never trusted the few who were truly kind, even well into adulthood, because I expected them to flip. The woman I refer to as my real grandmother passed away over two years ago, and I never fully trusted her. It's sad to me now that I know more about myself, and my life.

This is what I do know: I am not a sociopath. I am not an animal. I am a person. I am deserving of life, actual life. I was a child when those horrendous things occurred, and I survived it all because of my parts. I know that I actually am capable of human emotion, a fact I was unaware of until very recently. DID took a long, long time for me to fully accept. Logically it made sense to me, but I'm still working today to remove the damage done by detrimental people.

*

CHRIS ROBIN
Chris was diagnosed with 7
personalities in 2013 at age 49

I had no idea that DID existed in my life or the lives of others until the death of my partner and soulmate in December 2012. My entire world exploded and collapsed all at once. My family and friends advised me to get professional help, and through therapy for my grief and anxiety we found out that I have DID.

I have only begun my journey of learning about DID. I am just beginning to accept that trauma from my childhood created personalities as an escape from the hurt and pain. Over the years and various events that were traumatic, more parts grew because that was the only way I coped for dealing with what went on around me. I have begun to work on opening the lines of communication with my parts, and I'm learning more about them all the time. Some parts are quite young and communicate only with physical sensations and feelings, while other parts are children, teenagers and adults.

As a child I lived with an alcoholic parent, a parent who suffered from anxiety and stress, and an older sibling who was controlling and selfish. My adult situation has changed, but deep down inside these parts have held onto memories, feelings, emotions and physical sensations that have impacted my entire life.

The twenty-five years I spent with my partner, Beth, were secure, safe, adventurous, and loving, and unlike any other time in my life. Her unexpected death severely impacted me, and sent all my parts scrambling to make sense of what happened. I spent many years dissociating to help me cope, and breaking those habits has been difficult. Learning new ways to cope and communicate with my parts has been helpful and useful, and has opened my eyes.

*
QUINN ROSE
Quinn was diagnosed with 9
personalities in 2016 at age 21

I don't know much about how my condition came to be. My memory is pretty bad because of everything I went through. I don't remember much from my childhood except my family fighting for custody of my cousins who were abused by their mother. My uncle married a woman who had two other kids, and then they divorced and he left without a trace. I didn't get to see my cousins for three years, which was hard because for six years they had been like siblings to me. Skipping forward, I was in middle school when people started noticing changes about me. I became more aggressive and bullied others, even though I am normally the sweetest person you will ever meet. I didn't know what people were talking about when they told me of these events, but it got so bad that my mother pulled me out and home-schooled me.

It subsided a bit after that, until I started dating a guy who lived up north. I was only fourteen years old, and thought I was in love. He was sweet, funny, and got along with my family. It was Christmas and we were having a wonderful time. We went outside to enjoy the stars for a bit and even though my mother was efficient at keeping a watchful eye on us, he was clever in his schemes. This is my first recollection of abuse. I was raped by the person I I loved. He held me down and wouldn't stop. Ever since then, I've hated Christmas.

After a while he ended up living with me and my parents. I never told them about the rape incident. My family is very sweet and tries to help the less fortunate, and I know they couldn't handle the truth. It would crush them. But it kept happening throughout the time he lived with us; he would find clever ways. I blacked out through most of it. The next couple of years are kind of a blur. My sister married a guy she knew for only three months. He began to torment me, and still does. I then dated someone who was really abusive, both physically and mentally. I also met my best friend six years ago.

Only recently, at age twenty-one, have I learned that I have DID. I was at a hotel with one of my friends and boyfriend, and was a bit tipsy when the first personality revealed herself. Her name is Luna; she is the sex addict of the personalities. After that, everything in my life started to make sense: my strange behaviors, blacking out, memory loss, and strange stories people told me. My alters are as follows:

Raven: Controller, honest, sassy, and likes pin-ups.

Luna: Only likes to come out when I drink, and is a sex addict.

Trixie: Six years old, loves candy and stuffed animals; she is also highly advanced in the scientific area.

Carley: OCD, shy, timid, and loves to write poetry and cook.

Danielle: Boyish, likes to chop things, violent, defender.

Roxy: Loves cigarettes although I'm allergic. She always wears a leather jacket, doesn't believe my body is hers, and is psychologically destructive; a rebel, bully.

No Name: Depressive, loves to draw, and self-harms.

Yuno: Was created because of my best friend/boyfriend, and is the definition of nearly psychotic girlfriend. Literally Gasai Yuno.

Harley Quinn: Unknown yet, but, I will assume, is a lot like Harley Quinn. She uses the term "Puddin" a lot in her sketches.

*

AYA SAKURA
Aya has been living with 7
personalities since childhood

Before I start telling you about anything, I want to state a few things. First, I used to have a system of seven personalities including me, but now I've got a system of three personalities including me. My system currently consists of me, Brianna, and Clive. Sabrina, Makah, Lucy, Sayu, and Alice also used to be part of my system. I speak of Makah, Sabrina, Alice, Lucy, and Sayu in past tense because I consider them gone, though technically they've either merged or are in hiding and inactive at the moment.

While I'm a Dutch girl, Brianna and Clive (and Alice used to) consider themselves British. Lucy and Makah considered themselves Dutch, and Sayu and Sabrina considered themselves both Dutch and British. This means that the alters who think of themselves as British speak mainly English and have different mastery of the Dutch language, and vice versa for the alters who consider themselves Dutch.

Instead of talking about what brought on my condition, as I'm not comfortable talking about that, I'll talk you through my journey so far. To begin with, I'll tell you about myself. I'm Aya, a nineteen-year-old Dutch girl. I'm very introverted, sensitive, and not very confident. I study human resource management. I'm not assertive at all and

31

sometimes I can be very absentminded. I consider myself quiet, patient, and serious. I do have a sense of humor, though. I get told a lot that I'm helpful, ambitious and kind. I'm the main personality and the one who leads my life.

Clive is a twenty-year-old male with blue hair. He is the main protector of my system. He's very laid-back, gentle and caring, and emotionally very stable. Clive helps me to relax when I'm stressed. His job is to protect me from stress and stressful situations, and to keep me physically safe. He tends to be more extroverted than introverted, and is assertive. I mostly describe him as my inner self helper or the big brother I never had.

Brianna is female and also twenty. She's both a protector and persecutor. Brianna's responsibility is holding all my negative and bad emotions and memories. She keeps me safe from emotionally dangerous situations and specializes in keeping people away from me. She's extremely extroverted and assertive, with a lot of confidence. Brianna is, as she says herself, a lady, and will always act and move that way, while being completely potty-mouthed.

As long as I can remember I've heard voices in my head telling me about my surroundings and telling me what to do. When I grew older, I began having blackouts. After I saw Clive and Sabrina physically in front of me, I got scared of the voices and connected my blackouts to my voices. This happened when I was away on a week-long school trip in my fourth year of high school. I felt very uncomfortable and unhappy back then. I never saw my alters again after that trip. When I got home, I started talking to a school counselor whom I could trust and confidentially tell everything. He was quite concerned and after he talked once to Alive, he forced me to tell my parents about my others (as I like to call my alters).

I advanced to my fifth year of high school. The school recommended that my parents take me to mental healthcare. The psychologists at the mental healthcare office (MH-office) took half a year to examine me and figure out what I had. I hated the whole trajectory. During that time, every time my parents looked at me they were trying to figure out who was out, and what went wrong. That hurt me really bad. My mum disliked the MH-office and started searching for someone else to help. Makah and Sabrina merged around that time. I think that happened so they (Sayu) would have better control in and over the system.

Mum found a life coach and after a lot of hesitation I went there under protest, together with my parents. Because it felt better, I quit the MH-office before even getting an official diagnosis, and started talking to the coach who helped solve a few small things. I wanted to stop worrying my parents, and told them a few of my others had disappeared. Just before my final exams in high school, Sayu either hid or merged and I got a boyfriend. I stopped going to the coach and my parents finally calmed down.

The next six months were peaceful, but after I went to college everything escalated. I studied biology and medical laboratory research, and people there kept telling us we should share possible personal problems to keep everyone safe. So stupid me asked for a confidential staff member I could talk to. But he was also a member of some high council (I can't remember what) and used the information I gave him confidentially in that position. He thought I was dangerous in the lab, and after a lot of talking I was allowed to do practical work as long as I removed myself from the lab when I started dissociating. I went to one practical session, and was then told I didn't keep my promise. The directors forbade me to go into the school lab. When I needed lab time to observe real work, they said I could go because it wasn't in a university building.

The day I heard I wasn't allowed in the lab anymore, my boyfriend told Alice, "You can't come out anymore; you are dangerous." Alice suffered severe derealization; she was shocked and went into hiding. When I got home I told my parents I was quitting college. When asked why, I broke down and told them what was going on. My parents and I went to the university a few times to talk things over. The university wanted a security statement from a special psychiatrist saying that I was safe in a lab. I really didn't like this psychiatrist. In fact, I hated him. He had forgotten the first appointment, so we had a very short chat in which he immediately said that maybe I had been abused; my parents were sitting right next to me.

After a lot of struggling I finally gave up on my bachelor's degree, and Lucy also hid. I started working two part-time jobs, and again went to the mental health office. This time they spent almost a year examining me. I tried to divert the attention from my alters as much as possible, both at home and at the mental health office. They then said they didn't know, and sent me to my current therapist.

I lost almost all my social contacts that year. Around the time of the referral, my boyfriend and I broke up. Brianna completely blocked him. I quit one of my jobs. This all happened just before summer break. I then started my bachelor's degree in human resource management. I had to go on a trip with unknown people, which freaked me out. I wasn't able to make friends in my class and felt very lonely. For half a year I tried to transfer to another class, but that didn't happen. Eventually I became isolated.

Halfway through my first year I regained contact with a friend from high school. At some point I told her and her boyfriend about my alters. Her boyfriend is now a very good friend of ours. He was even able to get Brianna on a bike, something at which only Clive succeeded at before. In the last half year, I have made a few friends outside school.

A few months back, Alice showed up a couple of times. She still thinks it's 2014 and isn't in very good shape. Only Brianna has talked to her once or twice; Clive and I aren't able to. I don't know why she appeared again.

I got all the credits for my first year, and began my second year last September. My friends all went to study abroad. I was lucky and was put in a different class. I still had to go on another trip, which Clive did. He likes that kind of thing, so he enjoyed himself.

While in the first year of my human resource management program, I went to therapy. I don't talk about my alters there, because I'm scared they'll force me to tell my parents again, and there'll be severe consequences. I started group therapy sessions at the same office but am making no progress, so I'm now trying to feel safe enough to talk to my therapist about my alters. My goal now is to finish my bachelor's and to achieve communication with my system.

*

MATTHEW SANCHEZ
Matthew was diagnosed with 8
personalities in 2015 at age 16

My earliest memories are of my childhood home. It was me, my sisters, and my parents in our little house in the woods. We had dogs, a garden, and a big yard full of wildflowers—but we didn't have stability. My father was an alcoholic. He was loud, cruel, and abusive. Being so young, I could barely understand it. All I knew is that I was being hurt and there wasn't anything I could do about it. My only escape was nature. I would sit outside and daydream about a place where I could be happy, where I could sleep soundly without shaking in my bed when I heard my father stomp around and slam doors. I wanted a place where I never cried.

When I was seven my family moved to a new house with my grandparents. I thought that now that my grandparents were there, my dad wouldn't hurt our family as much. I was wrong. My grandmother was horrible to us. She pulled our hair, grabbed our arms, and yelled at us for being sinners. She insulted and criticized, and barked at everything. My father only grew more frustrated and drank more. The clearest memories of abuse are from this time. I can still remember how he looked when it happened; I cannot get that look out of my head when I think of him. My DID developed to cope with the heaps of trauma.

I lost time. Even today I can't remember parts of my childhood. Good and bad memories are lost forever. I couldn't remember things that people told me I did like incidents of pulling hair, screaming, and running off. I couldn't remember any of it. I was a very meek child and couldn't imagine doing anything like that to anyone. That's when I heard the voices.

When I would sit in my room, trying to remember, I felt resistance. I would get headaches and thoughts telling me, "Why remember? Why behave? Why care?" In my imaginary world that I now call my headspace, I began to meet the people who had been causing so much trouble. Their names were Bucky and Santiago. Bucky kept me company and always cheered me up after events of abuse. Santiago lashed out at people who hurt me, and sometimes at people who were trying to be nice. He really could never tell the difference between friend and foe.

Over the years, my home situation got slightly better as my mental health declined. My whole brain went foggy and I forgot about Bucky and Santiago. I fell into a horrible depression for years. I was constantly battling suicidal thoughts after realizing what had happened to me for so many years. When I saw a therapist in 2013, my mind started to clear and I heard the voices again. Santiago was back, but Bucky never returned to my headspace.

In high school, everything went bad. When needing to take notes, I would hallucinate and panic. To stop me from doing so, Santiago took over and did anything except learn. We both fought for control, and argued over health and grades. We never agreed.

I was losing time, weight, and sleep. I was so sick and depressed that I was beginning to seriously contemplate ending my life. Santiago begged me not to. He told me it was not the answer. I refused to listen to a voice in my head that had caused me so much trouble. Before I could succeed, Santiago told my mother of my suicide plan and got me into a hospital. He saved my life, and I know that I would not be alive if it hadn't been for him.

Santiago helped me to recover even further. He helped me recover from my eating disorder, my depression, and even helped me start my transition as a transgender. As my physical and mental health returned and stabilized, other alters came forth. Their names were Link, Davina, Regina, and M.

Santiago continues to save me from my mistakes and works with me to become the best person we can be. Together, as a system of functioning parts; working together.

*

FLOSS SCOTT
Floss was diagnosed with at least
4 personalities in 2016 at age 48

I witnessed abuse and I too was abused physically, mentally sexually, racially, bullied, threatened and much more. This started at the age of five. I was made to feel unwanted, the black sheep of the family; unloved and not good enough. As I grew up I was constantly rejected, but I am determined to do good with my life.

When I reached eighteen I got engaged to my first husband, whom I trusted and loved. He treated me like I was his everything. I bought my first house at the age of nineteen and sold it a couple of years later to upgrade to a bigger house. This was my security for when we had kids. Problems started when I had our third child. My husband lost interest in me and sought sex elsewhere. We worked things out for a short period and had our fourth child, but sadly he changed again and started behaving irrationally. I feared for my and my children's lives, so the police were involved. Our breakup came within a couple months of my mother's funeral, so I never had a chance to mourn her death. Something always came along to cloud everything going on, so I never really got the chance to deal with trauma that had happened in my life. My motto became "I'm going to pick myself up, dust myself down, and carry on bigger and better." I did this with anything bad, and never knew that it was my way of just shutting things out.

I entered into relationships but always ended them once the men became attached. When they brought up marriage, I'd be gone. I got engaged a few times, but ended the relationship before any planning started. I found that the guys I had relationships with chatted with other women behind my back, and so I would end the relationship. Eventually, eleven years on, I settled and trusted this one person and was having fun. But two years in, my health turned and I was constantly hospitalized with unexplained pains. My childhood seizures returned, and I was having problems walking. I was also having more blackouts, memory loss and chronic pain in my spine. Things went downhill rapidly. The seizures became worse, and so did the pain and side effects from both. Within twelve months I couldn't return to work and was never going to be able to drive again. This totally changed my life and brought the illnesses that were lurking in the background to the forefront. It's taken five years to be diagnosed with non-epileptic attack disorder and DID, along with nervous system centralization and chronic pain disorder.

When I spoke to a couple of family members and my kids about DID, it was no surprise to them. They said that they had always known I had different personalities. Thankfully it hasn't changed how they treat me or anything. But I recently remarried after nearly twenty years, and my current husband deserted me within a week of my DID diagnosis. He didn't want to deal with it. We had been together for eight years, and I haven't changed other than the illnesses that he's been dealing with for the past five years. So why would having a name for one of my illnesses make a difference? Well, apparently it does.

My three children and I have now been left to deal with all this alone, along with all the other traumas we've been going through lately. This breakup has totally broken me down to the bones. Some days I'm dusting it off, but other days I can't stop crying and asking myself what I've done to deserve this. I'm too ashamed to make it common knowledge, and so only my kids and my sister know.

I had to do some research on DID, as I hadn't heard of it before my psychiatrist mentioned it. On reading, I started to understand myself, which is something I had never been able to do before. I have five alters with names: three main ones and two child alters who are five and twelve. The three main ones have different jobs.

One is the calm, loving, and would do anything for anyone. One is the protector, provider, parent, and worker. One is the fighter.

They will appear when they need to, and change during the day depending on the situation and my needs. The child personas appear only after a seizure or when I'm feeling vulnerable.

I'm finding that this is life-changing for me and my family, because knowing all this is helping me to no end, and I'm determined to work on all my health issues and get the help I need to face it all. This process is in motion, thankfully. I'm very positive about this because I feel negativity breeds negativity, so I want to be positive that things will change for the better now.

*

PAULA SUNDWALL
Paula was diagnosed with dissociative amnesia in 2006 at age
36 and diagnosed with at least 4 personalities in 2014 at age 44

Something very bad happened to me before the age of five. I know this, not because I have a memory of the event or events, but because at age five I began wishing I could be reborn so I could be as innocent and happy as a baby again. My memories before that age are repressed, and so far I haven't found a doctor or therapist who will help me to unbury them.

During my childhood and adolescence I was molested by my Nana's two sons who lived next door. My memories of these incidents are fuzzy and full of shame. Aside from this, I have been raped twice that I can remember, though I did black out partway through each time. When I got divorced in 2001, my parents disowned me and I entered into yet another abusive relationship with a man who choked me. I ultimately moved out because he beat me up, in front of witnesses. I don't know if just the repressed memories were what caused the DID or if it was a combination of everything, all the accumulated abuse over a lifetime. Someday I hope to find out.

I'm actively seeking help, but am finding it very difficult to get mental health care providers to even believe in DID. I found a man who uses hypnosis to uncover repressed memories and then helps the client recover from the trauma, but he requires a doctor's note and I can't get any of my providers to write me the note I need.

*

KERRYJANE VOTH
Kerryjane was diagnosed with
35 alters in 2013 at age 53

I guess the hardest thing for me to do is to remember. Remembering is totally dependent on which alter is "online." It's the nature of DID to segment parts of our consciousness so that those most painful, life-threatening experiences can be blocked out so we can function in our daily activities. It results in a form of amnesia, affecting the person's ability to create an autobiographical timeline of his or her life. It's a protective mechanism that works really well under life-threatening circumstances, but becomes a disability when the threat is no longer present.

I have a hard time experiencing attachment to friends and family members, because attachment didn't happen with my primary caregivers when I was a very young baby. And because this attachment didn't happen, I wasn't able to experience the feelings of safety that are required to develop normally through my early years. It takes a lot to stop the normal development of attachment to caregivers with young children. It takes physical and/or emotional neglect, and abuse or medical trauma.

It isn't so important to me to know the details or to prove to others that this kind of severe emotional and physical abuse and neglect took place. A trusted relative confirmed those early years of neglect, and the parts of me who experienced the abuse remembers those events. The fact that I have been diagnosed by a psychiatrist using a specialized diagnostic test called the SCID-D test (Structured Clinical Interview for DSM-IV Dissociative Disorders), which is one hundred percent accurate in diagnosing DID. This is enough for me to know that my experiences did happen, and were severe enough to cause my brain not to integrate through the normal developmental stages that children should reach between the ages of six to eight.

It's unfortunate that children who experience this level of abuse are then set up by life to be abused further. This is the path that I was put on very early. The complete indoctrination into the church with no autonomy whatsoever, the added stresses of being a preacher's kid—it was like living in a fishbowl, along with the abuse and neglect by the parents behind closed doors that then, over time, were emulated by my sibling. This then became the norm as I moved out into the world with acquaintances and in my romantic relationships. It affected my ability to work and function in my daily life. And yet in spite of this, I did accomplish success with my children and myself.

I became a parent at seventeen years of age. I had my second child at age twenty-three, and the last child at twenty-seven, which resulted in the generational trauma being passed down to the next generation. This has been a tremendous cross to bear, since I became aware that it was being passed down through me even though I actively sought therapy and professional support at every step along the way while raising my children. To this day, I still see family patterns repeating themselves. Some are of my making and some not, which leads me to believe there may be a genetic component to the passing of trauma to the next generation.

I've been separated for the last seven years after being in a sixteen-year relationship, and a nine-year relationship before that (married twice). I'm single, not interested in dating, and probably never will because it's more than enough work to manage my poly- fragmented system. To be in a relationship with me would be like being in a relationship with a whole group of different people, some adults, some children, all at the same time.

My service dog, Dax, has been a great companion and support since coming to live with me in 2016. I did most of his training with Thames Centre Service Dogs. Dax is able to alert me before a switch with another alter takes place, sometimes up to five minutes before. This gives me time to prepare or to become aware of triggers to avoid the switch. He provides deep pressure therapy during episodes of derealization, dissociation and panic or anxiety. He has made it possible for me to go grocery shopping, run errands and socialize casually, which keeps my daily life moving in a more normal flow.

I still need professional support through my trauma therapist, occupational therapist, and advocacy through a case management worker with Canadian Mental Health Association. Having Dax along with the added professional support has made it possible for me to live independently. For all intents and purposes, if the casual passerby looks at me, he or she won't see anything untoward. My system is able to pass, as they say. It's only when someone spends time with me that she will start to notice differences in my behavior and memory.

Since coming into therapy, it's interesting for me to be living a life that is so new, that at times I don't know what to do with it. This sense of newness is brought on by the development of what the professionals call co-consciousness. It's really self-actualization, and is one of the most important aspects of developing cooperation and gaining memory and communication among alters. Without it, I experience my days much differently than those who are integrated and are conscious of their daily activities. If I'm not co-conscious and you ask me what I did today, the answer will depend on who is online at that moment. So you might get: all I did was sleep all day, or all I did was walk the dog several times today, or all I did was play on the internet all day. There isn't often a cohesive experience of doing all these things in the same day. So it can be frustrating to feel trapped, bored and unproductive and not understand why the body is so exhausted.

The reality is that I did all those things in one day, but suffered amnesia between the alters who were living out the activities. And because of the amnesia, I don't mark time the same way most people do. For me, time does not exist. I don't live my life in a linear fashion. Yesterday is today and vice versa. I can experience yesterday just the same as a day fifteen or twenty-five years ago. An hour can feel like a week, a week can feel like just a few minutes, a year can totally disappear. I call myself a true time traveler.

Through the trauma therapy that I started in 2013, I've been learning more about what dissociative identity disorder is, and is not. I've gained a deeper understanding of how trauma affects the mind, body and spirit, and I'm learning how to manage cooperation and communication among alters with mindful meditation, good sleep hygiene, financial hygiene, outdoor exercise, wholesome foods, and human contact. The most important healing part for DIDs is learning how to have healthy attachments.

I've been working through the trauma memories using motor sensory psychotherapy with a trained specialist to heal the body from complex posttraumatic stress disorder. Not everyone who has PTSD has DID, but most of those with DID have PTSD. Even so, I still find my littles (young alters) insisting on trying to deal with adult responsibilities, which makes for very difficult situations while out in public. It's all a matter of learning, communicating, observing, tolerating, and safe exposure over and over and over again to teach the body that it's truly safe now, and that we can "adult." I'm learning to map my system and to identify each alter by name.

I'd like to leave you with this description that my system wrote about itself today. I hope you enjoy it.

Let me tell you what it's like being a DID system:
….we are like
individual
flickering
sparkles of sunshine on the water.
each undulating between
consciousness,
unconsciousness
and co-consciousness...
a never-ending shifting
of knowledge,
skills
and
abilities.
with waves
derealizing
then
depersonalizing
and dissociating
as they break upon the sands of life
that keep wearing off our rough edges.

The Other Side of Midnight
BY SUNSHINE

On the other side of midnight while most are asleep
lies awake a girl, can't you hear her weep?
She walks about the house calling out my name
no one else can hear her, to them we're just the same.

She stands in front of a mirror afraid of what she'll see.
She leans in a little closer, and questions "Is that me?"
Her eyes are sunken in and her look is dark and cold
once where laid such beauty, age has made her old.

Wrinkles taken over, scars across her cheek
where abuse has left its mark, and the toll has made her weak.
Her hands are frail and crippled, leaving her with little strength.
Her life hasn't been easy, and the world has not been kind.

Once dark and beautiful flowing hair, now so brittle and untamed,
she holds her face in her hands, feeling so ashamed.
Her legs are so unstable, her feet are bare and worn,
her clothes no longer fit her, dirty, tattered and torn.

She huddles in the corner; can't you hear her cry?
How could this have happened? When did life pass her by?
She walks from room to room, like she so often does,
searching aimlessly about for a glimpse of a life that was.

Her anger is not to be reckoned with,
her screams a piercing sound,
this goes on forever it seems, until what she's lost is found.
I am the one who sees her, look closely can't you see?
It is I who stands before you,
it is her that is me.

*

CHAPTER TWO

Learning the Diagnosis

It is a great mystery that though the human heart longs for truth, in which alone it finds liberation and delight, the first reaction of human beings to truth is one of hostility and fear. -ANTHONY DE MELLO

Digesting the diagnosis can bring a flood of emotions that vacillate like a rollercoaster—accepting one day and angry or denial the next. Or we may even pretend we never received such a diagnosis. What was your reaction when you were diagnosed with dissociative identity disorder?

*

ADRIANNE ALLEN-LANG
Adrianne was diagnosed with 10
personalities in 2015 at age 18

Receiving my diagnosis was a huge weight off my shoulders. I finally had confirmation that it wasn't bad memory, and that I wasn't a liar. I still don't have support from my parents. My father pretends it doesn't exist and my mother just refuses to speak about it, and makes it a habit to call my alters by incorrect names. The few friends I have were good with it, but I never spend enough time with them for them to fully understand what dissociative identity disorder is.

*

GAIL BUSWELL
Gail was diagnosed with 13
personalities in 2002 at age 24

When I got my diagnoses it didn't come as a surprise. I always knew I was different. I had my quirks and nobody understood me. I was very isolated and withdrawn. Being able to put a name to what I was experiencing was a huge weight lifted from my shoulders. Being able to research it and reach out to others who also had DID was a real lifeline for us.

*

KATT HART
Katt was diagnosed with hundreds
of personalities in 2011 at age 20

When we found out we had DID, before the diagnosis, at first we were comforted to know that there was a name for what was happening. But it didn't take long for the discomfort and fear to kick in. The denial got very bad for the main alter who was around at that time. That denial and fear lasted on and off for two years; it was awful. Eventually, when we started to feel more comfortable with that idea, we sought a diagnosis and it was very validating, very comforting to know that we weren't making things up. It was a great feeling knowing that's what was definitely going on so we could finally find ways to recover and improve.

*

ROSEMARY HAWKINS
Rosemary was diagnosed with at
least 5 personalities in 2014 at age 46

At first it was a relief that I had some answers to the massive amount of confusion and doubt that I felt within myself. To have a label meant something I could grasp. This very quickly turned to rage, however. I felt cheated! It wasn't fair. I missed out on so much. I felt like my life lay in pieces and that I would never be able to make sense of who I was. I asked myself, who are you? I seriously didn't know, and I certainly didn't trust myself. I struggled with a lot of anger, and that quickly turned into depression as I began to understand the impact that DID had on my life.

I didn't tell my family. We were all still struggling with grief, and I didn't want to burden them with a diagnosis that I didn't even understand myself. I also felt embarrassed and didn't want to admit to anyone what was really going on inside me. I went to great lengths to hide it, and I also spent a lot of time hiding from myself. I felt utterly alone! Completely damaged beyond repair, and somewhat of a freak! At first I didn't want any information, because I was scared of what I might find out. I didn't want to know. I had a very good psychiatrist and a wonderful psychologist who luckily supported me initially.

*

AMELIA JOUBERT
Amelia was diagnosed with 12
personalities in 2013 at age 15

When I found out I had DID, my first thought was relief because I finally had a name to put to my experiences. It finally made sense that

I heard people talking in my head and I couldn't remember days on end. My second thought was extreme fear, because this disorder comes from trauma. At the time I was identified with having DID, I didn't remember any of my trauma. Before being diagnosed, I didn't mind the others, even considered them friends. But the thought that I could have gone through some trauma as a child that I had no memory of terrified me and seemed impossible. It led to denial, and as trauma memories started to surface, I didn't know how to handle them. I tried to ignore the other people I share a body with, and used alcohol as a way to do it. By age fifteen, I had driven myself into alcoholism.

Eventually I was hospitalized and put in an inpatient treatment facility where I began to accept that this was my situation and there was no changing it. Things then got better. In this facility I began to remember more details of my trauma, and this time I actually dealt with those memories in a healthy way. All the work I did in that facility and since has led to my having a great relationship with my alters, and coping with my past in better ways.

*

AMANDA LINEBACK
Amanda was diagnosed with hundreds
of personalities in 2013 at age 31

I had been in the deep depths of depression, dissociation, and several suicide attempts for about two years before I was diagnosed with DID. I saw my first therapist two to three times a week for a little over a year. She was the first person I ever trusted to talk to about any of my hidden struggles. I worked on my self-image, learned how to stop the negative feedback loop in my head, and finally began to open up so I could release my hidden pain. She helped me realize that I had a very distorted opinion of myself and what healthy relationships and attachments are supposed to be like. I learned I didn't have to feel guilty for saying no, and that boundaries are not selfish. On the outside I was going through the motions of life as if I were feeling better. In reality, I was still masking my true feelings and numbing my pain with anxiety medicine. I continued to lose hope and began relying on unhealthy coping mechanisms to release relentless emotional pain. I began to plan my demise and knew I needed help.

I went to Brentwood Meadows, a behavioral hospital, and was admitted to inpatient care. After three months of inpatient stays and a few months of outpatient therapy, I was stable enough to be at home. I was diagnosed with obsessive-compulsive disorder, complex PTSD, major depressive disorder, anxiety, panic disorder with agoraphobia, body dysmorphic disorder, and ADHD. I was prescribed medication and then more medicine to keep the side effects of those medicines at bay. While in Brentwood Meadows, I made an appointment with a therapist who specialized in eye movement desensitization and reprocessing (EMDR). After a few minutes of normal chitchat, the therapist had me take the Dissociative Experiences Scale, a screening test. After he got my score he made an appointment for me to see his colleague who specialized in dissociative disorders.

On September 25, 2013, I met Dr. Dawn Gable and was diagnosed with dissociative identity disorder. It shattered everything I believed about myself and forced me to discover the truth about my existence. It was so weird because even though I hadn't changed a bit, I felt like an alien in my own body. I felt ashamed, alone, and apathetic. I was also angry because I wanted a normal life, and I knew that I had a lot of work to do. My body was frequently numb and my head was dizzy. At times, I couldn't speak and time went missing. I wanted to be able to take some medicine and move on with my life. I had already worked hard just to make it to this point and I was tired. I was so tired of fighting to exist that it was hard to force myself to breathe.

*

JANE MACDONALD
Jane was diagnosed with 3 personalities in
2014 at age 35, and currently has 6 alters

It's hard to put into words the emotional turmoil that came with my diagnosis. It wasn't my first mental health diagnosis, but it was one of the most devastating. This isn't to say that I was happy about any of the other diagnoses, but with most of them I had already self-diagnosed and wasn't surprised to have them confirmed. However, with DID it was a different story. I didn't know much about this diagnosis other than the basics which were covered in my college psychology classes and what I saw in the media, neither of which were particularly helpful. Although I now know that I exhibited many of the classic symptoms, I never would have thought to apply this particular label to myself. To me, DID was something that happened to other people. I think one reason for this was that the stigma associated with this disorder in particular is still so prevalent and I didn't want to admit that I could possibly have something that severe. Whatever the reason, the diagnosis hit me pretty hard, and it is still something I am coming to grips with almost two full years later.

I think the best way for me to describe how I felt is to liken it to the stages of grief one goes through when you suffer the loss of a loved one, but with certain key differences. Although I had most of the emotions of a traditional grief reaction, I didn't always experience them in sequence. Sometimes I would skip a stage and return to it later. Other times I would experience more than one stage at a time. My emotions often were, and still are, a complete jumble. I can feel sad, angry, ashamed, and other emotions all at the same time. Some days I was or am fine with the diagnosis, and other days I am in complete denial. It is very overwhelming. Today, I have more or less accepted my DID and the fact that I have others living inside me, but that doesn't make it any easier to deal with.

At first, I remember feeling completely overwhelmed. I had already received multiple psychiatric diagnoses and wasn't thrilled to have another one to add to the ever-growing list. I was angry that I hadn't recognized the symptoms in myself first, since I am a psychology graduate. This anger increased when I found out soon after being diagnosed that a previous psychiatrist had noted in my file that I had dissociated while in his office and an alter came out, a fact that he never once mentioned to me. This was a full seven years prior to my official diagnosis of DID.

I also experienced a great deal of confusion. Did this new diagnosis void the previous diagnoses? Did this mean I no longer had, for instance, borderline personality disorder? The two diagnoses manifest themselves in a similar way. So was I replacing one label with another? Or was this in addition to the other labels, in which case I had yet another to add to an already alarmingly long list of mental illnesses? To be saddled with yet another diagnosis when you already have eight others can be devastating.

Sometimes I would tell myself it didn't matter, it was just one more. Just another label. I have never been much for labels, finding them more stigmatizing than helpful. Other times I thought, "Oh gods, another one! I am so screwed up. I will never be normal." I was also uncertain about exactly what this diagnosis meant. Was it a life sentence? Was it something that could be treated with medication? Is it something I would recover from, or something I would have for the rest of my life and just have to learn to live with?

Unfortunately, my psychiatrist didn't provide me with any information on this new diagnosis, so I was left to do research on my own. I tried to stick to reputable journals and articles, but those are hard to come by online. Thankfully, I found online support groups for those living with DID. I learned a lot from conversing with people in these groups, but still found it confusing. My experiences didn't always match those of others. Would I grow to be more like them as I came to know more about my others, or was I just different? If I was different, did that maybe mean that I didn't have DID at all? It's natural to compare oneself to others with the same diagnosis, but it is also problematic because there are so many different ways DID can manifest itself. It was very overwhelming and confusing. Over time, I have learned to accept that my DID experiences may be similar to others or different from theirs, but it is still an equally valid diagnosis. I am also learning to stop comparing myself to other people.

Anger has figured prominently in my life since my diagnosis of dissociative identity disorder. A lot of this anger stems from learning that a previous psychiatric determined that I had not only dissociated in his office, with one of my alters coming out, but also that I scored high on a scale used by clinicians to diagnose DID in patients. What angers me is that neither of these facts were mentioned to me by said psychiatrist and I found out about them only recently from my current psychiatrist who was reviewing my files, seven years later. Why had I not been told? Why would such an important fact be kept from me? Why did I have to wait seven years for someone to find this buried in my file? I could have been treated for this and maybe have had a much better handle on my alters had this psychiatrist bothered to tell me or to refer me to someone who could help me with it.

I continue to struggle with this diagnosis. There is some comfort in finally having an accurate diagnosis of my condition. Without one, it is difficult to research and learn about my illness or receive proper treatment. However, I still experience a great deal of fear. It is still a very highly stigmatized and highly misunderstood diagnosis which is not portrayed accurately or favorably in the media. Because of this, I have kept my diagnosis a secret from my family and majority of my friends. This makes it incredibly difficult to find any kind of support, except from people who also have DID and are in the same online support groups as I am.

I had to tell my employer, as she has seen me switch. While she tries to be supportive, I know that she does not fully understand what is happening. I worry about certain "others" coming out at work who are more destructive. I also fear my coworkers finding out and judging me. Many times I still feel completely alone with this diagnosis. It is not something I can talk about openly with my friends or family. It is something that I feel I have to keep secret.

On any given day I still experience a wide range of emotions surrounding this newest diagnosis. It frightens me that others might find out about my condition. I feel sad and overwhelmed to have yet another diagnosis. I am angry that I wasn't diagnosed earlier. The fact that most research indicates that DID is something you live with for life, that it cannot be cured, can be very disheartening. I am grateful that I know what it is. I am glad that I have an excellent psychiatrist who is helping me. On good days, I feel like I can learn to live with this but on other days I am not so optimistic. Other days it is a real struggle. For better or worse, it is who I am and what I will have to learn to live with.

*

CRYSTALIE MATULEWICZ
Crystalie was diagnosed with dissociative
identity disorder in 2015 at age 29

I still remember the day I was diagnosed. I was heavily dissociated and when I finally grounded two hours into a therapy session, I remember hearing these words: "I think you have dissociative identity disorder." I didn't cry. I didn't get angry. I just sat there on my therapist's couch, completely numb to emotion. Part of me already knew the diagnosis. It wasn't the first time I had heard it. Therapists had asked me about it before, but I brushed it off and a discussion never went any farther. But my mind knew the diagnosis was right. I knew what DID was from my studies in psychology, and felt that it fit a lot of what I had been experiencing for so long. My heart, on the other hand, didn't want to acknowledge the truth. I knew what having DID meant. I knew the diagnosis meant I would have to acknowledge my trauma. It meant that I had to acknowledge that I had been abused every day by the very people who were supposed to love and care for me. I wasn't ready to admit all of that. It was much easier to live in denial: denial of the abuse, and denial of my DID.

In some ways, the diagnosis did bring me a sense of relief. I have always been a very analytical person. When I don't know something, I research until I find an answer. I like solving things. I like answers. And here was my answer. Here was the solution. Here was the name for what was happening to me. I had been in and out of the mental health system for nearly fifteen years at that point, and received over a dozen diagnoses that included mood disorders, depressive disorders, anxiety disorders, attachment disorders, and personality disorders. I had taken countless medications: antidepressants, mood stabilizers, anxiolytics, and antipsychotics. None of them seemed to work. Therapy hadn't worked. Of course none of it worked, because none of it acknowledged the DID. You can't help a patient with diabetes by treating for irritable bowel syndrome. The same goes for mental health. Nothing was working for me all those years, because I was consistently being treated for the wrong things.

Some of my diagnoses were accurate and still affect me. In addition to DID, I also have PTSD and persistent depressive disorder.

A lot of the symptoms of my dissociative disorder were mistaken for symptoms of other disorders. What appeared as changes in mood was not bipolar disorder, but rather different parts coming through. The lost time and disconnection with reality was not psychosis, but rather symptoms of dissociation and derealization.

Within a few weeks of being diagnosed, I bought a dozen books on DID. I wanted to know more than the very minimal facts I had already learned in college. I bought books written by psychiatrists, and books written by people with DID. I wanted to learn as much as I could from all sources. In a way, I went into reading wanting to prove my diagnosis wrong, but instead I ended up resonating with so much of what I read that I found it difficult to deny my diagnosis.

The first few months after my diagnosis were up and down. On some days I was able to accept my DID. I wrote a lot about my experiences, which helped me work through all the chaos in my head. Other days, however, were not so easy. I would tell myself that it was all just a big mistake, and that I didn't have DID. Whenever my therapist mentioned it, I shut down. Sometimes I even said out loud, "I don't have DID today," as if I had a switch somewhere that allowed me to turn the disorder on and off at will.

I experienced a whirlwind of emotions. Anger, because I knew the reason I had developed DID was due to the people who had hurt me. Fear, because I didn't know what I was in for, and I was scared for my future. Anxiety, because I didn't know how the outside world was going to treat me. Worry, because I didn't think my peers would accept me. Sadness, because the diagnosis felt like a tremendous loss.

I was diagnosed one month after I ran away from home. In order to protect myself and my safety, I had to cut myself off from everyone in my old life. I was living in a new city where I didn't know anyone. I hadn't developed trust with anyone aside from my therapist, whom I was seeing a couple of times a week. I ended up seeking support online. I wrote about my DID in my blog, and connected with others who shared the same diagnosis and the same experiences. I joined DID groups on social networks in hopes of connecting with people who understood. I had a group of close online friends who were supportive of me as well. Even so, I still longed for support in the outside world.

Some months after my diagnosis I finally opened up to people in my life about my DID. I was offered a job writing for a mental health website. At first I had no idea that I would be writing about DID. I was still getting used to the diagnosis myself, and didn't think I was ready to be open about it with thousands of people. After a lot of back-and-forth, I took the offer. My name was forever connected to DID. I knew people would find out, so I decided to come out of hiding. I had deactivated all my social media accounts and was living off the grid when I ran away. I told my friends and acquaintances, both old and new, what was going on.

I didn't know how everyone would react but, to my surprise, they were all supportive. Some were not surprised by the diagnosis. My coworkers were continuously supportive of me, even on the days when I struggled, even though they didn't quite understand what was going on. I finally started to lose the shame I had carried with me for so long, and the shame I felt when I first received the diagnosis.

*

ALICIA PETTIS
Alicia was diagnosed with 40
personalities in 2015 at age 16

I was fearful of what others would think. Living in a household where the outward appearance is worth more than what's truly going on made me terrified to ask for help or even a diagnosis. I kept it to myself and my friends for a long time. The internet and library books were the only resource of information I could obtain. They were also easily hidden from my parents, who would put me through hell before accepting that I suffered from any disorder.

*

SUNSHINE PURCELL
Denise was diagnosed with 17
personalities in 1995 at age 30

I was angry and confused. I had never even heard of such a thing. I told my therapist she was wrong. I went out and bought the Diagnostic and Statistical Manual of Mental Disorders to read and prove her wrong. I was scared, because I didn't know what this meant or what would happen. Was I crazy? How can someone's mind do this? What caused it?

I was given the book *Trauma and Recovery* and when I read it, it was like someone was describing my life to a T. The hardest part is believing that someone could hurt a child in such a horrific way that there was no alternative but to "go away" in order to deal with the situation. I couldn't quite talk about what happened, or say that something had happened to me. It was always the feeling that it happened to someone else. The only comfort I felt or feel was that it was a normal response to an abnormal situation. I wasn't crazy. It wasn't all in my head. The voices, the feelings, depression, mood swings, other names that were familiar but I had no idea why.

My family didn't know what to say, and of course they didn't believe me, because then they would have to admit that something did happen and they did nothing about it. They didn't do anything like get me therapy when it happened; my whole system was malfunctioning in order to survive. The more trauma I incurred, the more personalities were created. When something happened to me, my mind would search to see if something similar had already taken place and whether a personality was already formed. If so, they would attach the memory. If it wasn't similar, then a new personality was created to handle it. Denise, my birth name, was fractured. She doesn't exist except by name only, and sometimes by outbursts. I am the one who fronts the most. My name was "Me," but to make it easier I chose Sunshine. I don't have friends. We have a big trust issue, and it's hard to have friends when no one understands what my personalities are and why they happened. My family knows I have it, and another relative has also developed it—same circumstances, different person—but we don't talk, so it doesn't come up.

*

ERICKA REEVE
Ericka was diagnosed with over
25 personalities in 2013 at age 26

I'm not even sure, honestly. It was a few various things and then I was just "gone." Again. I don't remember the specific day or where I was. I know my current doctor diagnosed me. I know how I feel about it now, but when I was diagnosed she was speaking to one of my parts without realizing it. I hadn't actually met her until nearly a year into our therapy. At that time I was terrified. I knew I went to doctor appointments pretty frequently, but did not know specifics. It sounds goofy, crazy, but it is what it is.

My doctor had begun to explain things at that time. One of my parts, A (she prefers not to use her full name), finally told my doctor she was speaking to Trixie and not me! That threw things off a bit, but we worked together and figured it out. I'm coming up on three years into my diagnosis, and I still find it terrifying.

I do not have much support. I have one friend who actively speaks with me and we, and openly. She does not fear them and tries to understand the best she can. My husband finds it frightening and exceptionally difficult to accept, even though we've known each other for many years. He struggles.

*

CHRIS ROBIN
Chris was diagnosed with at least
7 personalities in 2013 at age 49

Emotions are probably the hardest part of dealing with my acceptance of having DID. I learned all my life to compartmentalize my world—that was how I was able to survive and function. Feelings and emotions had their place, and most of my life was spent not feeling anything. When the love of my life—who lived with me for half my life—died, all the compartments blended and I spent well over a year just going through the motions of trying to find a new normal. When I began to wake from that numbness, with the help of my therapist I began to realize that I wasn't alone in my mind. She began to point out and explain what might be happening to me. It exhilarating to know that I wasn't crazy, but it also was the scariest thing I've ever had to face about myself, and I had to learn to face it alone.

How could I share this with family and friends? I couldn't and still haven't been able to share with anyone but my therapist. She shared her insights, read books and articles, and has explained to all the parts of me in a way they could understand, what is going on in my mind.

I spent months denying that I had DID, while at the same time feeling glad that those voices in my head that were so familiar were more than just my internal instincts. Everyone acts differently in different places and situations, but when I realized that I was doing more than that, and at times I couldn't figure out what was real and what was not real, and how I lost time or couldn't remember interactions, I began to believe that she might be right: I have DID.

It's taken me well over a year to begin to accept that I have DID, and it has helped ease some of the tension within myself. Looking back, I can remember being defensive and argumentative about the thought of having DID, while at the same time having a sense of comfort and relief that there was a reason why I act the way I do. I think that at some point at the beginning of my journey into learning to live with DID, I felt every emotion possible.

*

QUINN ROSE
Quinn was diagnosed with 9
personalities in 2016 at age 21

The first time, my memory got erased by my alters. The second time it was revealed, I felt dread and fear, also sadness and anger. Why is this happening to me? How can I deal with this? Who did this to me? Why?

*

AYA SAKURA
Aya has been living with 7
personalities since childhood

My first emotions after learning that I was living with DID were panic and denial. At first I was almost paralyzed by the shock. After I calmed down a little and was over the first shock, I began to deny it. I told myself I was just forgetful, that I could not have a disorder. Every time I didn't notice anything from my alters, I thought, see? There's nothing wrong with me. But when I began to see the connection between blackouts and my voices, I panicked. How would I ever get control over them and my life? One of my biggest fears is losing control, so this was terrifying. After that I began to learn about everyone in my system just to understand myself, my selves, ourselves.

In a sense, knowing I had something which was a disorder meant knowing I wasn't crazy, because others had this condition as well. I had support from people I met online. Some of my friends broke off contact with me, but others became even better friends, and they support me as well.

*

MATTHEW SANCHEZ
Matthew was diagnosed with 8
personalities in 2015 at age 16

I felt an incredible amount of relief. I had been living with so many people inside my head, and I had no explanation. When my therapist opened her book and told me what I had, I felt like I wasn't alone. My close friends, family, and girlfriend all know about my DID, but my girlfriend is the only one interested in being kind and understanding to my alters.

*

FLOSS SCOTT
Floss was diagnosed with at least
4 personalities in 2016 at age 48

When I first learned I was living with DID, I couldn't wait to get home and read up about it. I remember being in the taxi, and I googled it straight away on the twenty-minute journey home. At first I seemed okay, but within a couple of days it started to sink in, and that's when the fear and upset began. I was relieved to be able to speak to someone who had been diagnosed with something similar just a year before. I was more concerned about:

Roughly how long would it take to come to terms with?

Did people treat him any differently?

How did it make him feel as a person?

How did it affect him emotionally?

After having some answers to my questions and a two-hour conversation about how it was making me feel, I felt that I could handle this. In the days ahead I found I was distancing myself from my children and spending more time in my room, getting upset uncontrollably. This went on for a few days, and then I would be fine, and then crying again out the blue, but it had been worrying me inside. I told my husband that the one thing I feared was that he would leave me and not want me anymore. A few days later he did just that. He told me he didn't want to be with me anymore. I'm now divorcing him. I really didn't expect this after being married for only six months.

*

PAULA SUNDWALL
Paula was diagnosed with dissociative amnesia in 2006 at age
36 and diagnosed with at least 4 personalities in 2014 at age 44

Even though I was initially diagnosed with dissociative amnesia, I consider that to be the time when I was diagnosed with DID, because I knew that it was more than just amnesia. I had, by then, become accustomed to upsetting things, and knew well how to push them to the back of my mind and not think of them. My counselor said we would work together to learn how to deal with the PTSD that surely precipitated the dissociation, but we never did. I steered every session into harmless directions, and she allowed me to. We were both to blame.

It is only now, eight years later, that I am beginning to deal with the truth of my disorder and genuinely trying to find ways to deal with it. There are people in one of the online support groups that I belong to who say that it is not so much a disorder, but a choice that your mind makes in the face of terrible adversity. They are proud of their "others" and are integrated into systems that communicate with each other and follow rules and just generally get along. I am jealous. For me, it is a disorder. When I get caught shoplifting with no memory of how I even got to the store (my license was revoked after four unremembered accidents) that's a disorder. When I lie down to take a nap and wake up to find that all my medications have disappeared, that's a disorder. My life is chaos. Sometimes I want to die.

*

KERRYJANE VOTH
Kerryjane was diagnosed with
35 alters in 2013 at age 53

I experienced complete horror, fear, denial, anger, surprise, smugness, dissociation, flashbacks, flight, grief, and more after I learned I was living with DID. My only knowledge of DID was what I had watched from the TV show "The United States of Tara" and "The Three Faces of Eve." Both, I came to learn, are highly exaggerated and sensationalized Hollywood portrayals of DID.

It was only through the education and emotional support provided by my trauma therapist that I was able to start to understand and begin to accept this diagnosis. It was also through this education that I was able to learn a language to be able to talk about what I was experiencing within my body.

*

*

Artwork by Andre
Denise Purcell's alter
www.sisterdiarieswithsunshine.com

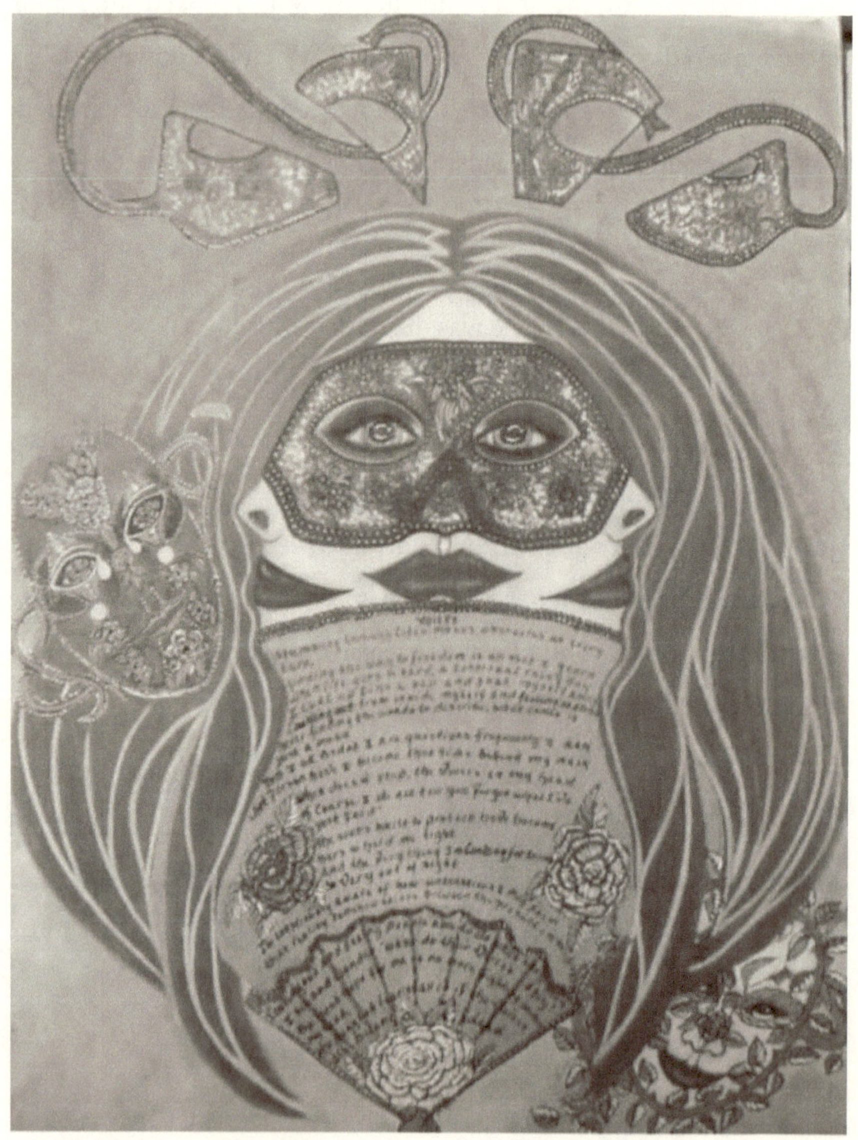

CHAPTER THREE

Awareness of the Others

At the heart of personality is the need to feel a sense
of being lovable without having to qualify for that
acceptance. -PAUL TOURNIER

Self-esteem, identity, and body image are closely related. They are also deeply woven into the fabric of our being. Yet when one is composed of many parts, at what point do we become aware of our dissociative identity? What about family and friends?

*

ADRIANNE ALLEN-LANG
Adrianne was diagnosed with 10
personalities in 2015 at age 18

Prior to my diagnosis I was aware of my DID, but only of Adrian, not the others. Adrian and I would talk all the time, and even he would get confused about blank spots in our memories, as we had always been co-conscious with each other. I first figured out something was wrong when I started having massive gaps in my memories, things being done that weren't done before, coloring ins, cleaning, homework, etc. It was a scary experience, because I didn't know what was what. I started to speak about it when I was nine but was quickly shushed by family and professionals who said I was just seeking attention. It wasn't until I was fifteen and speaking to a psychiatrist about what I was going through that he suggested DID, and everything clicked into place for me. My family swears they never noticed anything funny, but you'd expect that, with DID being a chameleon disorder.

*

GAIL BUSWELL
Gail was diagnosed with 13
personalities in 2002 at age 24

Prior to my diagnosis I was weird. I kept to myself, but was happy. I had no friends, but I think this was more of a defense mechanism. We desperately wanted friends, but lacked the social skills to maintain friendships.

*

KATT HART
Katt was diagnosed with hundreds
of personalities in 2011 at age 20

We found out the name for it when we were eighteen. Our host alter at the time knew about the voices, accusations of doing or saying things they didn't remember, finding possessions they didn't buy, and finding writing and drawings they didn't do. But before finding out there was a name for this, they didn't know what exactly was happening. Friends and family kept reporting changes, things that were out of character, a lot of remarks similar to "I don't know who you are any more." A lot of people knew something was happening but had no idea what it was, or why.

*

ROSEMARY HAWKINS
Rosemary was diagnosed with at
least 5 personalities in 2014 at age 46

I had no idea. It was a complete shock. I spent all my time disconnected from myself. I was so disconnected that I did not recognize any changes within myself. I had spent all my adult years in this state, so I didn't know of any changes in my personality. Looking back, I can see small differences which were signs, but I didn't know of them at the time. There were times when I felt afraid for no reason, rebellious and angry for no reason, and times when I couldn't account for periods of time. I never looked into any of these occurrences, though. I was too busy running from myself and staying disconnected to notice. My DID started when I was so young that it is almost like I didn't know life without it. I didn't know any differently.

*

AMELIA JOUBERT
Amelia was diagnosed with 12
personalities in 2013 at age 15

When I was younger I didn't know I was any different than anyone else, but as I got older I began to realize that not everyone had other people in their heads. I knew I was different; I just didn't know what it was. For a while I even thought I might have ghosts possessing me, because I didn't have any other explanation. I had heard of multiple personalities but I didn't know much about it, and the wrong information I did have, saying people with multiple personalities didn't know they had other personalities, so I assumed I didn't have it. Of course today I know that information isn't true. My mom told me she did notice things that she knows today were my alters, but at the time they just confused her. She said she would always get very confused because sometimes I would randomly start talking with a Southern accent or like a child.

*

AMANDA LINEBACK
Amanda was diagnosed with hundreds
of personalities in 2013 at age 31

I was unaware that I had DID prior to my diagnosis. Until I knew differently, I thought I was experiencing things just like any other person. I have always heard the different voices in my head, but I thought they were my conscience. I have always had a really hard time making decisions. I would get high anxiety when it came time to answering questions, because I would have so many different opinions. I would get overwhelmed and not know how to answer. I would think that no matter what I answered, it would somehow be a lie because of the disagreements going on in my head. The voices in my head have been there as far back as I can remember. I thought of them like the little angel and devil on people's shoulders like they showed in the cartoons. I thought that everyone had their own internal voices who gave different opinions on everything.

*
JANE MACDONALD
Jane was diagnosed with 3 personalities in
2014 at age 35 and currently has 6 alters

Prior to my diagnosis I was unaware that I had dissociative identity disorder. I was aware of the symptoms that I had, sure. But I didn't know enough about DID at the time to put two and two together and realize that was what I was experiencing. Since I was a young child I had felt like I was often a completely different person in different situations. I know that everyone feels somewhat different in various situations and at different times, but this was more than that. This felt like a complete shift in my identity. Normally I was a very timid, shy and introverted person. I didn't speak to many people. I had a lot of anxiety and was frequently depressed. I preferred to stay inside by myself rather than socialize. Yet in some situations I became quite the opposite: I would be social, outgoing, and self-confident.

One such situation was when my dad took my sister and me on vacation every summer, and some winters, to visit a bed and breakfast in the countryside that was run by friends of ours. It was more than just feeling more relaxed or at home with my friends; it was like I was a completely different person. Even my family commented on this. I know now that this is because Jess, one of my younger alters, was the one who was out while I was there. Jess is playful, outgoing, and has none of the anxieties or low moods that plague me most of the time. She also came out at other times in my life. She mainly came out when I was with my father and we went on adventures and hikes in nearby nature areas and hiking trails. At other times I became angry, rebellious, and disrespectful for no reason at all. I know now that this is what I am like when Angela, my angry teenage alter, is out. At other times I would be terrified, cowering in fear in my bedroom or hiding under the covers for no reason. At first I dismissed this as panic attacks, but I felt differently than during a normal panic attack; younger somehow. I have learned that this is how Clara, my mute two-year-old alter, often is.

Besides noticing changes in personality or identity, I also noticed other things that I couldn't explain. In high school I started to feel as if my body wasn't my own, as if I were a small child trapped in a body that was too large for me. I often got the sensation that my hands, in particular, were too big. I never quite knew what to make of this, but it scared me. I was scared enough that I didn't mention it to anyone, for fear of how they would react, likely dismissing me or telling me I was crazy.

I noticed other things as well. I would find pieces of writing in my journals that were not in my handwriting. I would lose time, sometimes just a few minutes but at other times a few hours. I usually put this down to not paying attention, having a bad memory or just zoning out. I also was aware that I had very few concrete memories of my childhood, particularly before age eight. Again, I dismissed this as having a poor memory. It never occurred to me that I might be blocking out anything or suppressing some kind of trauma. A part of me thought it was normal to forget my early childhood. I was a kid, after all. So yet again I didn't think much of these or my other symptoms.

Other little things would happen too. I would find clothes and other possessions in my room that I had no recollection of purchasing or receiving as a gift. Again, things that I didn't know quite what to make of, but was too scared to tell anyone about.

Then there were the voices. I remember hearing them as a child but figuring they were something like an imaginary friend. Feeling ashamed, I felt the need to also keep this a secret. This only got worse as I got older. In high school I started to become interested in psychology. I remember a fieldtrip we took to a psychiatric hospital where we did role playing to teach us what it was like to live with severe mental illness. One such role-play I was involved in depicted a woman who was hearing voices telling her to do things. This terrified me. Although my voices were different than the ones in the role-play, I quickly came to associate hearing voices with schizophrenia, and therefore with severe psychosis. That was certainly not a label I wanted to have, so again I kept it to myself.

As an adult, I recall having an appointment with a psychiatrist and having the voices get louder and louder, and more and more difficult to ignore. I tried to communicate to him what was going on, but I wasn't able to do it in an effective manner, and he seemed to completely ignore what was happening. He was only interested in treating me with medication for my anxiety and depression. DID wasn't a part of any of my current diagnoses, so it was ignored.

The first time I was introduced to the concept of dissociation in any meaningful way, it was in a treatment program for personality disorders. It was presented to us as a form of zoning out, similar to when people are driving and forget how they got from one location to another. It was explained as a symptom of borderline personality disorder, which was one of my diagnoses at the time. I accepted this explanation, could identify that I frequently dissociated, and finally felt like at least some of my symptoms were able to be accounted for. Identity disturbance, as they call it, was another trademark characteristic of borderline personality disorder, so I figured that my alters or others were just a part of that. I didn't think to ascribe the symptoms I had been experiencing to anything else. I thought my new personality disorder diagnoses covered most of what I was dealing with, and I was happy to have an explanation for it at long last. Even if the explanation didn't cover everything that was going on, at least it covered some of it. Any explanation, I thought, is better than none, so I latched onto it. It wasn't until a few years later while seeing my current psychiatrist that I officially received a diagnosis of DID, and that came only as a result of one of my alters coming out during a therapy session.

I'm grateful to have a name to put to all these symptoms now. It is scary and frustrating, but at least I know what it is and why I was experiencing the things I was. It is frustrating that I didn't figure it out earlier. It also angers me that my previous psychiatrists never clued in, but I know that not everyone in the psychiatric community accepts the legitimacy of DID as a diagnosis. Although it can be overwhelming, it is better, in my opinion, to have this diagnosis and to begin treatment as soon as possible.

*

CRYSTALIE MATULEWICZ
Crystalie was diagnosed with dissociative
identity disorder in 2015 at age 29

I wasn't entirely aware I had DID before my diagnosis. I always knew something was off but I could never quite put a name to it, and neither could the plethora of mental health professionals I had been to for over a decade.

My symptoms really started to be apparent in adolescence. My demeanor changed, often for no reason. My therapist believed it was the mood swings of bipolar disorder, but I didn't think that was right. If anything, I was consistently depressed, never happy or even remotely content. I just felt different a lot of the time, like I was not myself. I couldn't recognize myself as myself. I knew it was me, but I didn't feel like me.

I lost time as a teenager. When someone asked what I had done the week before, I often couldn't remember. Even when I tried to, I couldn't remember any of my childhood. Nothing bad, but nothing good, either. I knew that I existed as a child, but I just didn't understand why I had no memories. It was incredibly frustrating.

I self-injured with no recollection of ever doing it. My psychiatrist believed it was psychosis related to bipolar mania. The medications never worked. I still lost time. I still felt so disconnected from myself. I started drinking and using drugs to cope, but that only made things worse. When I started hearing voices, I thought to myself, this is it, I am crazy. At that time, the only people I knew who heard voices were people with schizophrenia, the ones you hear about who are locked away in hospitals. I didn't think I was schizophrenic, but not knowing what DID was at that time, I didn't know what was wrong with me. They don't teach about DID in schools, so I never had any idea.

My opinions changed so rapidly in ways I didn't understand. I'd put an outfit on, only to feel compelled to change it several times. As an adult, I would buy things and return them the next day, unsure of why I bought them in the first place because they were not things I would normally buy. I'd look in the mirror and not recognize that it was me.

I struggled a lot with my identity. At times I didn't feel like a girl. It wasn't a typical identity confusion that teenagers can experience; this was different. I would go through periods when I didn't feel like I was in the right body. I didn't want breasts, so I tried to hide them by taping them down. I hid my body in baggy clothes. But then I didn't feel like that anymore. The confusion was gone, but only temporarily; it always ended up coming back.

I had moments when I felt like my real life had frozen. I would reach a point when, for whatever reason, I couldn't handle certain things so I retreated into myself. On the outside it appeared as if I was just daydreaming. On the inside, I was hiding from danger.

Because of the environment I grew up in, I didn't have any genuine input from family, as we only saw them briefly on holidays. I didn't have any friends outside of school, and as an adult, the only people I interacted with were the people I worked with, at a job my mother and I shared. My mother regularly called me crazy and said I was mentally ill. She told everyone that I was severely bipolar, a compulsive liar, and that I could not be trusted. But that was more of a way for her to control me than it was an honest assessment of my mental health. Unfortunately, her actions kept most people from getting close to me, which prevented them from recognizing that there was a problem.

When I finally told a close friend about my diagnosis, he didn't seem surprised. He said he had even met one of my parts before. I never even knew, as he never said anything. He said my behavior would change and I would start to act like a child. I would cry a lot for no reason, and just wanted to color or play, so he let me. He said it was all just part of who I was.

*

ALICIA PETTIS
Alicia was diagnosed with 40
personalities in 2015 at age 16

I noticed that I began losing time and not remembering things I had done when I was in seventh grade. When I didn't lose time and stayed conscious, I noticed that I would become enraged at the tiniest thing and my voice dropped slightly. Sometimes I felt like curling up in a ball with a stuffed animal and taking a nap; my voice would be chipper and high-pitched like a little kid. On those days, I kept to myself because it terrified me to talk to anyone besides my friends. My friends were the ones who informed me of my alters in seventh grade. They told me about the mean and always angry girl, Sophia; the little girl named Kayleigh who liked tutus, the color pink, and anything soft; and the silent depressive one named Kyle who liked self-destructing.

*

SUNSHINE PURCELL
Denise was diagnosed with 17
personalities in 1995 at age 30

I knew I heard voices. They didn't tell me to hurt anyone or do anything. It started out as voices fighting in my head, and I knew it wasn't me or my thoughts. I was thirty. I had terrible mood swings. I would be fine one minute but the next minute would feel miserable or depressed. I had so much turmoil within my head and my whole being. I experienced feelings I didn't have a reason to feel, but sensed and reacted to them anyway. I had no logical reason for losing track of time and wearing different clothes and things.

I didn't feel as if I belonged anywhere. I didn't know why I was alive, and pretty sure that I felt like I wanted to die. I just wanted peace and quiet. There is always talking in my head, thoughts that are random and make no sense to me because they aren't mine. My family, my parents, thought I was just a miserable, ungrateful child who was always wanting attention. The funny thing is that I hate being the center of attention. I hate crowds. I hate interacting with people. I hate compliments. And I hate not knowing from one second to the next what my body will do, my mind will think, or my mouth will say.

I have nightmares and always did, flashbacks about people hurting me. I have body memories when certain parts of my body will remember a trauma, even though my mind doesn't, and will react to it. A trigger, smells or visions, pictures, movies, talking about it all bring bad stuff up.

I have sleep disturbances, depression, isolation, flashbacks, anger, no self-esteem, depersonalization and seizures caused by the emotional part of the brain called pseudo seizures. I take anxiety medication but it doesn't help. Antidepressants don't work for me; they tend to make me incapable of thinking or feeling anything, or they work backwards in my system. I have information and lots of books on dissociative identity disorder, but they don't help much.

It's confusing to me how the world works, why people hug and how people can experience good feelings, because I can't feel much of anything, let alone think I might do good or be worth something to someone, even my children. They know now and think it's pretty cool that I have people in my head. They all have a relationship with my alters, as does my fiancé. They have gotten to know each one and have found gifts in them. My parts have many talents.

I am in therapy and have been for twenty years. We work on symptoms, depression, cognitive behavioral therapy, and some eye movement desensitization and reprocessing therapy, EMDR. It's a crapshoot, because we are all different and not something out of a textbook. The best way to know about it is to learn from someone who lives it every day, trying to balance the real-life things from our real-life things. People get scared or don't believe in it, but it's real, and really hard. It affects our health like stomach problems, headaches, seizures, social skills, eating disorders, relationship problems, and wrong diagnoses. It's not something we can just get over, or we would have already. I would do anything for anyone, because I know what it feels like to hurt. And the worst part is that sometimes when I meet someone who really clicks with me or one of my alters, they get scared off when they find out, or I become a project to them. I believe they should have the chance to decide if they want me as a friend. I don't really expect they would, because it takes patience and understanding, but it could be rewarding if you take the chance. All we need is love, and we can give love.

We didn't choose this, so we shouldn't be cast out like we have the plague. We're dealing with consequences from someone else's actions. A lot of those people won't suffer any consequences, and they will never know how they have affected our lives in every way, every day. As many times as I give up, I go on, because I am worth it. We are amazing people. Just take a chance. Strength comes in numbers; we are many.

*

ERICKA REEVE
Ericka was diagnosed with over
25 personalities in 2013 at age 26

This is a bit tricky. In high school it was an ongoing joke among people who knew me better than most, that I had multiple personalities. The "Umm, who am I talking to?" Or "Are you *you* today?" Questions and jokes were pretty regular, or so I'm told. I don't have many memories from my life prior to the last five-ish years. I'm nearly thirty, by the way. My family was very much oblivious, and still is, to the frustration of my parts (alters).

It has been pointed out to me on several occasions that I wasn't myself yesterday, or today, or whenever the case was. All that I had really become aware of was that when I got angry, unpleasantness occurred. I would black out, as I began calling it, and wake up in random places, even different cities or states. I actively began trying to reduce stress and anger because I knew that when that occurred, I would not remember anything. Nothing. Nada.

*

CHRIS ROBIN
Chris was diagnosed with at least
7 personalities in 2013 at age 49

I had no idea that DID existed prior to my diagnosis. I knew that I compartmentalized my life. I knew that work was work, family was family, friends were friends, and so on, and they just don't mix or mingle. I knew that I was unsure and uncomfortable in social situations and that I had a hard time understanding the world. When I met Beth, she became more than just my lover. She became my confidante and interpreted the world for me, and I found myself in situations where I could finally be all of me at once. Where all the parts of me worked together and I could be a teacher by day, unionist by afternoon, and family and friend on the weekend. In between, I could share all those parts with one person who accepted me for being all that and more. Life then was livable and manageable. So when she died, that all ended.

Suddenly work, family and friends blended and I lost the control to separate them. Friends and family noticed differences at times, but I don't think they ever really thought of it as multiple personalities. I have spent so much time dissociating my life that I do it pretty well and it goes unnoticed. I'm just now beginning to recognize it myself. I am getting better and finding it easier to recognize when I dissociate, and at least know that I am doing that even though I still can't stop it. I am learning to ask for help and to find friends around me who can bring me into the present.

*

QUINN ROSE
Quinn was diagnosed with 9
personalities in 2016 at age 21

I haven't told my family. They are in denial about a lot of things, and we haven't yet revealed anything to them. My friends, though, took it with open arms and actually kind of knew about it.

*

AYA SAKURA
Aya has been living with 7
personalities since childhood

Prior to starting therapy, I was partly aware of my DID. I was aware of a few other people protecting me and helping with daily life, and I was experiencing time leaps, as I call my blackouts. Around that time I heard the voices of others in my head who were giving me tips and telling me things about myself or others, or just about my daily life. I heard six voices in my head, each with its own characteristics and things they would tell me. One voice, Sabrina, always told me I should care less about everyone's opinions, and that the feelings of others weren't my problem. Another, Makah, would help me make important decisions. They all had their field of experience. They would help by telling me answers in class or on exams. Or they would tell me that somebody was angry with me and why. Basically, they just kept my life together and told me enough to keep me up to date so I could function.

I really didn't notice my blackouts then; I just thought time had passed really quickly. Memory loss was due to my thinking of some thing else and not paying attention to my surroundings, I told myself. For example, Alice, the one who was very sporty and enjoyed physical stuff, took all my PE classes and everything related to that. When I was in the changing room, she would come out and take PE. I only knew that PE always went by very quickly without really noticing or knowing that Alice came out. By the time I came back, I was in my normal clothes again and on my way to my next class. This phenomenon also happened when I felt panicked, sad, angry, unsafe, very tired, or when I just couldn't manage to go to school.

My friends and family actually did not notice anything weird about me. I think that is because my others (as I like to call my alters), are very, very cautious about other people finding out about them and always acted like me, or kept quiet. The reason could be that I absolutely do not want to stand out in any way.

*

MATTHEW SANCHEZ
Matthew was diagnosed with 8
personalities in 2015 at age 16

I isolated myself for the majority of my adolescent years. My family didn't see it as different personalities, just moodiness. My girlfriend was the first to notice that I wasn't acting like myself. My protective alter, Santiago, was not fond of my girlfriend. He was overprotective and worried that she would hurt me. She noticed that he would act colder than I could, and asked me about it. Reluctantly, I explained to her about Santiago's existence. She was incredibly supportive, and has become close friends with many of my alters.

*

FLOSS SCOTT
Floss was diagnosed with at least
4 personalities in 2016 at age 48

I spoke to my children straight away about being diagnosed with DID, and they said, "Mom, we already know you have multiple personalities. You just won't accept it." Well, I was totally shocked by this, but I've now accepted that I have DID. I then had to pluck up the courage to tell my sisters. When I made the phone calls, again I was shocked that they too thought the same as my children. When I asked why they hadn't said something to me, they said, "We just accepted that that's you, and we're not going to treat you any differently, as this is how we know you." I've not spoken to my friends about it, as I don't really want it going any farther, and they might tell others.

*

PAULA SUNDWALL
Paula was diagnosed with dissociative amnesia in 2006 at age
36 and diagnosed with at least 4 personalities in 2014 at age 44

Nobody was ever aware of it, to my knowledge. When I was nine, I asked my mother if I disappeared but still looked like me, would she come to find me? That seemed to me like some foresight into things to come. The problem was, I began drinking heavily at around age twelve and always drank to black out, so alters could have been making appearances without me or anyone around me knowing about it. Of course I was acting strangely; I was wasted. My first noticeable blackout that wasn't drug or alcohol-induced occurred a few months after I quit drinking in my thirties. I also experienced fugues, amnesia, and was hospitalized twice with no knowledge as to who or where I was for over twenty-four hours each time. Maybe somewhere deep down I had an inkling. I read *Sybil* as a child and was very aware of the things to look for. It's just that for the first twenty years of looking, the signs weren't there.

*

KERRYJANE VOTH
Kerryjane was diagnosed with
35 alters in 2013 at age 53

I was not aware of having DID before being diagnosed. I always knew there was something wrong with me, something that was interfering with my being able to function well with the everyday responsibilities of life. I was very frustrated and just couldn't understand why I was so intelligent and gifted in so many areas, yet wasn't able to do the things I wanted to do, or maintain stability emotionally. My family took great delight in reminding me, whenever they got the chance, to tell me that there was something wrong with me. They called me crazy and said, "There is something wrong with you." But no one ever said, "Hey, let's find out what's going on and help you to make life better."

I was blamed for the way I was, and blamed for whatever that something wrong was. The people who enjoyed being my friend were people who were okay with accepting me just as I was. I have been able to have several good friends over the years.

*

CHAPTER FOUR

Our Different Parts

In this universe and this existence, where we live with this duality of whether we exist or not and who are we, the stories we tell ourselves are the stories that define the potentialities of our existence. -SHEKHAR KAPUR

Living with dissociative identity disorder means that each personality exists as part of a group sharing the same body. Some of the personalities are related or the best of friends. Others don't communicate at all. How well do your personalities know each other, and how well do you communicate?

*

ADRIANNE ALLEN-LANG
Adrianne was diagnosed with 10
personalities in 2015 at age 18

My personalities know one another fairly well. Kitty (age four) and Pumpkin (age two) are the best of friends and spend a lot of time with Allie, who they call mum. Everyone talks a lot unless they're in another room of the inner world; they can't communicate through walls. We've come a long way since everyone came out of hiding. Muscle and Keegan used to bully everyone a lot and hurt the body, but we stopped that by finding outlets for them and everyone else, and currently they're all pretty happy.

I don't have control as such; they're their own people, but I can stop them from controlling the body in low-stress situations. But the moment I start to become too stressed, scared, traumatized, etc., I begin to dissociate, and someone appropriate for the situation will jump out and deal with it to protect me. And then while out, he or she will do some things for themselves (ha ha).

*

KATT HART
Katt was diagnosed with hundreds
of personalities in 2011 at age 20

The alters are separated into groups, and those groups can talk to each other and be friends, but the ones outside those groups can't, so that's something we're working on. A lot of the groups seem to get along with each other and work together, but there's some that cause problems and even hurt other alters. The alters try to protect each other from the ones causing damage and try to help those alters change their ways, but it's a lot of work and some aren't willing to listen. We have very little control over switching to different alters. Sometimes we can resist, but most of the time it happens anyway. We don't make an effort to hide ourselves around most people, though. Most of us don't mind if other people know about it. We only really try to hold back switching when it feels very negative or if someone is very triggered by something and may come out and start crying or lashing out at people.

*

ROSEMARY HAWKINS
Rosemary was diagnosed with at
least 5 personalities in 2014 at age 46

Because I am still so new at recognizing my alters, I still have a hard time knowing which one of them is around. I would have to say that I often don't know when each of them is forward. Having said this, though, I think it would be fair to say that they do fight at times. I have become aware of an internal dialogue between my five-year-old and one of my older alters. The older one calls the younger one a baby and makes fun of her. The five-year-old then sulks. It feels totally normal to me to have multiple conversations and interactions going on inside me at any one time. I am getting better at recognizing who is calling the shots at any given time, and the more I identify who is currently in control, the weirder it feels.

*

AMELIA JOUBERT
Amelia was diagnosed with 12
personalities in 2013 at age 15

I know the other main eleven alters who come out very well. We are a family and we protect and love each other. There are others who don't really come out, and we call them insiders. Some I know very well, and others I have never met. The main twelve of us get along well for the most part, but fight sometimes. We fight like family because we are family.

*

AMANDA LINEBACK
Amanda was diagnosed with hundreds
of personalities in 2013 at age 31

I am made of a system of alters who have their own subsystems. I would describe it like an extended family. The immediate extended family is the first system. Then those people also have their own system of alters. There are a lot of children and teenagers in my fronting or immediate system. I have between thirty-five and forty alters in my front system that help me get through day-to-day life. The decisions they make are based on the locked systems deep within. We love each other most of the time.

Big Manda: I am the one who is typing right now and am the vessel for most of us.

Baby: She sucks her thumb.

Little Amanda: She is four and she has a teddy bear named Hope. She is shy and gets scared easily.

Blonde Haired Girl: She is three and doesn't feel emotions.

Lola, Lily, Lila, and Maxx are siblings.

Lola: She is three years old and loves to talk. She loves to play. She really likes drawing with the outside kids, Jaylin and Jaden.

Lily: She is seven. Her favorite color is blue. She loves to play prize claw and eat Laffy Taffy.

Lila: She is also seven. She was created when Lily went away for telling secrets.

Maxx: He is eight and loves to eat. He loves dinosaurs. He loves to eat like he is a dinosaur. Mr. Chad bought him a nerf gun for his birthday, and he loves that too.

Jilly and JoJo: They are ten-year-old twin sisters. They have bright red hair and green eyes. Jilly thinks her mom is perfect and loves her more than anything. JoJo cries because she thinks she doesn't have a mommy.

Tyler: He is six and likes to play videogames. He likes to play Mortal Kombat with Jaden, because they are best friends.

Maria: She is nine years old and is quiet.

Sebastian: He is a very intelligent eleven-year-old boy. He helps the littles with big words and teaches them cool facts.

Katya and Sara are best friends.

Katya: I like to play tricks and keep outsiders as far away as possible. I am sixteen. I am tough, stubborn, silly, and smart. My best friend is Sara. She is the same age as me but she is so naive. I take care of her so she doesn't feel sad. I like boys and hip-hop music. I like to drive fast. I love to have fun, be wild and free.

Sara: I am sixteen years old and I am quiet and reserved. I am awkwardly shy. I trust people without their having to earn it, because to me everyone is good. I like to help others, because it makes people like me. I feel sad and depressed most of the time. The world and people in general disappoint me. Katya is my best friend and she keeps people from taking advantage of me.

Lauren: I am twenty-two years old. I tell things the way they are and remain unbiased during conversations. I usually come off cold, because I don't sugarcoat what needs to be said.

Nervous Diana: I am nervous and apprehensive about going places. I don't like crowds or people standing too close to me. I am always aware of my surroundings and keep us from being harmed.

The other teenagers are Sam, Sammy, Samantha, Stephanie, Michelle, and Carly.

Amanda: I was the host for us for most of our lives. I am a perfectionist, and anything less than perfect is useless. I was the room made of glass. I made decisions carefully so no would know anything about us. I delegated positions from inside so that we maintained our cover. I made sure we excelled at everything, and if someone needed to be created then I made sure it happened. I am fragile and delicate; the inner workings of the basic need to feel loved. I was shattered the day we were discovered, the day when the nightmares took over and Self-Mutilator took revenge on us. The nightmares caused Guilt to take over and then we were punished by Mutilator.

Demon: I am the ultimate protector. I come out when faced with life-or-death situations. I was made so we are protected from violence. I am the sum of all the hate, rage, and anger we collectively feel for the people who have harmed us. I have no fear, and I feel no pain. I am smart and tactile in my decision-making.

Self Mutilator: I punish the snitches for treason.

Guilt: I feel everyone's guilt and shame.

Wolf: I sense fear and can feel danger in my bones. I feel bad people when they are near. I can sense when someone is lying or being deceptive. I know when someone is being manipulative.

Lioness: I am the protector of the outside children, Jaylin and Jaden. I have witnessed every good and bad experience, which I use to make intelligent decisions. My job is to keep the children from any kind of harm. I make sure that the children come first no matter what, and can override anyone who is fronting in order to keep the children safe.

Gloria: I am an inner-self helper. I make sure we get to the doctor and take our medicine.

The Numb One: I shut off everything and everyone.

*

JANE MACDONALD
Jane was diagnosed with 3 personalities in
2014 at age 35, and currently has 6 alters

A lot of people with DID whom you will read or hear about will tell you that they have an inner world where their personalities all interact. Many have systems that they refer to affectionately as a gang, group, family, troupe, or collective, and have developed rules and guidelines that each member follows. Several will tell you that they have developed a system of harmony and cooperation among their alters, and that although things are still difficult, the key is their communication and coordination. In my own experiences on online support groups, I have found that many, even the majority, of people describe these types of situations.

Unfortunately, my DID experience seems to be vastly different. Mine is more like a group of strangers who all happen to inhabit the same body and mind and who, most of the time, are isolated and have little to no communication or even awareness of one another. To be honest, I am jealous of those who have developed cooperative systems. I suppose that would be my goal, but right now I just don't see it happening.

There are six alters in my system. I can identify them by age (well, most of them) and gender, but other than that they have no discernible roles, such as mother or protector. The exception is Kali whose age is unknown but who seems to be an introject of an abuser or abusers, and who tries to harm and kill the rest of the alters and myself.

Among the alters, only a few know of one another's existence. Angela, the teenage alter who is always angry and acts out, is aware only of Clara, the two-year-old mute alter. Emily, the eight-year-old, and Jess, the four-year-old, are aware of each other but none of the others. Clara is aware of both Angela and Kali, of whom she is afraid. Kali, as far as I can tell, is aware of Clara and Angela but not Emily or Jess. In the past I had Jack, who was aware of Angela, Clara, and Kali, but he hasn't been seen or heard from in many months. My psychiatrist feels Jack may have somehow merged with Kali, as they were or are both introjects.

Life with my alters is pretty chaotic. There is no harmony or cooperation. There is no communication among my different personalities and each comes out when and where they want, and for however long they want or need. Each one is out to serve his or her own desires and needs. I am only occasionally aware myself when one of my other personalities has been out, usually gleaned from writing, clothing, or what other people tell me.

There is no sense of a system or community, of friendship or family, or even mutual awareness. As you can imagine, this is very frustrating and can make life quite difficult. I have made attempts to communicate with my alters by leaving notes or treats for them, but no effort has ever been reciprocated.

The little I know about each alter I get more from a feeling when they are out, or from what my psychiatrist describes when he encounters one during an appointment. I envy people who have a sense of harmony and cooperation among their personalities and I aspire to someday achieve this, but for now it feels like every man or woman or child for themselves. For now, it is all I can do just to function and survive each day.

*

CRYSTALIE MATULEWICZ
Crystalie was diagnosed with dissociative
identity disorder in 2015 at age 29

My parts existed in chaos for years, because I didn't really understand what was going on. It was like a daycare full of children of all different ages. There were no rules, no organization in place, and the teachers had given up and left the building. That was what my system was like for such a long time. I am now starting to work with my system better, so our life doesn't have to be a consistent state of organized chaos.

For a while I didn't really care to take control. It's a lot easier to just dissociate and let another part handle things rather than trying to work through difficulties myself. I let my parts come out whenever they wanted, because I was too tired and emotionally drained to insist on taking charge. This ended up hurting me more often than not. I realized that I needed to step up and take some control. First, I needed to work on accepting that my system existed at all. As much as I was dissociating, I was still in denial that I had DID. Admittedly, this is something I still struggle with sometimes, but I'm getting better at acceptance. I also knew that I needed to work on staying grounded more, and encouraging my parts to explore the inside world, while I stay busy working on our life in the outside world.

My system is not so simple and organized as other systems are. I have a lot of parts. Some of my parts make themselves known. They have names and specific tasks in the system. Then there are parts who are not so distinct. A lot of them don't have names. I also have parts who feel like me, but aren't really me. There's a lot going on that I am still trying to understand.

I have a dominant part who knows the other parts in the system. He is sort of the self-proclaimed leader, making sure no one on the outside gets too close and that other parts don't reveal too much to the wrong people. He does get overprotective at times, especially regarding therapy. He can be a bully to the others. I let him know that he doesn't have to be in charge of everyone, that I can work to protect myself and the others. We are still working on a more balanced way of working together as a team.

A lot of my younger parts are close in age, and are close with other young ones in the system. They tend to stick together which helps them feel not so alone on the inside. I also have a part that doesn't acknowledge that he is a part at all; he believes he is the one and only. As far as our system knowing everyone inside, I think there are varying levels of awareness. It's sort of like a neighbor-hood where you know others live there, but you don't necessarily know anything about them. Some you know personally, others you don't even know their names. Some you talk to, others you don't. It's complex. There are disagreements between me and the other parts of the system, as well as disagreements among the parts themselves. Humans have disagreements all the time, and alters are no different.

*

ALICIA PETTIS
Alicia was diagnosed with 40
personalities in 2015 at age 16

My alters have a saying: they're the C.A.O. system, or the Chaos and Order System. At other times things are chaotic and harmony is out the window. Other times things are in order and everyone is working together and getting along.

It used to just be chaotic when I was a young middle school student who felt like I was crazy for even thinking I had such a disorder. Dealing with Sophia being angry and wanting to fight everything that crossed paths with her, and Kyle, who loved self-destructing with the closest object, was definitely a challenge. Control was the hardest thing I learned, and I have to relearn it again. Even though when I was younger I was able to control the switches and fight them back, now I can only put up my fists and pray that I can stay in control if I really need to. My alters grew in numbers, so it became hard to control what was going on. All my personalities are aware and know each other very well. They've also allowed me the opportunity to see and meet everyone, unlike when I was diagnosed. Some hid in fear that they might push me over the limit, since my mental stability wasn't all that well. Now, even I know all of my own parts.

*

SUNSHINE PURCELL
Denise was diagnosed with 17
personalities in 1995 at age 30

My personalities know each other and can interact with one another but not with me, Sunshine. I am out for the most part; I am the host. I see to everyday activities the best I can. I don't have control over any of my personalities. They emerge when they wish. For the most part, the younger alters, Sarah and Abbey, ages five and seven, come out. They are very strong willed and vocal which only stands to reason, since DID stemmed from them and a baby, Isabelle. They are out every day to play or watch television. They like to color and play marbles, fly kites, learn about planets and animals, and love whom they love dearly. They know they have one body, and they know they can't always come out and do kid things like see Santa, play with other kids, or talk freely in public, although they do slip up and get excited and become loud. They love doing things for others and are so considerate of other people's feelings. However, they also know my thoughts, and at times will reveal my thoughts without understanding that it could cause quite a mess of things. They have stuffed animals and act just like their ages. They have their own voices and ailments. Not everyone feels the same things, physically or mentally, at the same time.

The Smart One takes care of important things like medical appointments and dealing with insurance companies. She also has activities she likes to do, such as reading or researching. She's very good at getting adult things done.

There are two poets, a man and a woman. They come out to journal and write poetry. They don't have names and they really don't talk much.

I have an artist, Andre, who comes out to draw.

Boots is a party girl who can be very blunt.

Kasey with a K is a valley girl who likes having fun.

An older Irish man with a brogue is kind of the watcher of things.

Laura and Dale are teenage sister and brother.

Rachael is a teenager.

The Mother entertains and makes everyone happy. She looks like Donna Reed from the 1950s era.

There is Denise, and Isabelle, who is a baby with a blanket and who cries.

Charlie doesn't do much, but if things get out of control he offers solutions that aren't always in the best interest of anyone involved, but that's his job.

I sometimes forget to mention someone, and I apologize for that.

We don't have contracts and we don't have agreements, except not to hurt each other or anyone else. I have had scenes in stores when someone was triggered by something, maybe someone looked like our abuser and started crying. I only come to when they are done. I don't know how long, or what or who was out. I don't remember anything, and find out only if someone tells me or there is evidence. I could be doing dishes while Sarah is talking. So that's a weird combo.

I'm still just getting the hang of this, and I'm now more accepting of them. They saved my life. I don't ever want them integrated into one. That would feel like I lost a limb or a loved one. We just have to learn to work together. It's a long process, because they all have their own feelings, wants and beliefs, and they are all different. And then I have my own.

They say that we lived in fight-or-flight syndrome, always prepared for the worst. Everyone did his or her job. When I got older and the threat of those things diminished, they still were left with the memory, mostly secret memories that are locked up for protection. Now they are left with doing what they want. If you don't acknowledge or accept them, they can cause quite a mess with wrong choices, awful consequences, missing objects; those are a few. One day I hope there is a better awareness and under-standing. It's no picnic for us. The only quiet I sometimes get is white noise.

*

ERICKA REEVE
Ericka was diagnosed with over
25 personalities in 2013 at age 26

For the most part, they all are pretty familiar with each other. They work harmoniously sometimes when absolutely necessary, but most of the time they just don't bother. They seem to be trying, now that we're working on co-consciousness. Sort of.

This has definitely changed since I've been in therapy. I've seen countless doctors over the years, but for whatever reason this time it stuck—and she saw them. I think I really need to give credit to one of them. She's the one (the only one, really) who consistently attempted to get help. Because of her and a few others, we found this doctor who has been a huge asset to us.

I rarely, if ever, go out in public. They do that, but again we're currently working on it. So as far as control over them goes when in public, the answer would be none to hardly any. Jynx, for example, is the social one. She goes to the parties and events. Another will go grocery shopping and clean or do the boring events. I can barely function in my home, let alone venture outside.

*

CHRIS ROBIN
Chris was diagnosed with at least
7 personalities in 2013 at age 49

I am just learning to understand my parts. Some know each other really well and have communicated among themselves for years. Other parts are very much separate from the others and we are just now learning to bring them together. It has been difficult for the younger parts and the adult parts to communicate and understand each other. One part definitely wants to take control and have power, while others are timid and shy. Some parts are confident and others aren't.

There are arguments and disagreements among my parts, and that creates stress and discomfort, but my therapist and I are trying to work on opening clearer and educated communication. The goal is to get all the parts of me to work together and realize that at some time in my life that part was important and valuable. It takes a lot of mental energy to keep all the parts of me contained. For now it is easier and functional to have only some parts out at a time. So at work a few parts work together to help me work, while the others stay tucked away. Then in other situations, other parts take over to help, and so on.

With help from my therapist I've been able to create a house with rooms and floors, so every part of me has a place to be separate and comfortable when not needed. The house has a speaker system so that everyone can hear what's going on and can participate if they need to, and we have a conference room where we can talk and communicate. It's a weird process, but it's making things easier and better. We can now learn more about each other. I have been able to control letting them all out at one time, especially in public. I have learned to remove myself from situations where I can't control parts of me so that it won't be noticeable. That creates isolation and many private meltdowns. I have to learn to reach out for help now that Beth, my partner, is no longer in my life. That has been very hard to learn to do.

*
QUINN ROSE
Quinn was diagnosed with 9
personalities in 2016 at age 21

They are aware and can converse with each other. I have yet to meet them myself. I am left out all the time.

*
AYA SAKURA
Aya has been living with 7
personalities since childhood

That is actually different for every personality. In my current system of three, I know the names of my alters, their roles in the system, and what character traits they have. These are just facts, and I don't know them very well personally. I really do want to know them, so I'm working really hard on achieving that through mailing, talking to them and asking questions when they are co-conscious.

Brianna and Clive, however, know each other very well, personally as well as their function in the system. They are married in the inner world and have had a relationship for ages. They know exactly how the other would react and almost always are able to predict the actions of the other. It has been this way for as long as I can remember. I don't know how well Clive knows me on a personal level, but I do know he's very good at acting like me. I don't really know what that indicates. Brianna is very good at reading my emotions, and in knowing how I feel and why. So I guess she knows me pretty well, even though I'm not talking to her very much. I asked a good friend who knows all of us quite well. She told me that both Clive and

Brianna mostly know what I'm up to. My friend said they know exactly what I need in any given situation, which is to be expected, since they are my protectors.

When I had a system of seven, everyone knew who existed and what their names were, but not everyone knew the roles of the others, or who they actually were. All my alters, and I as well, talked to just a few others. Some had better communication than others, and some of my alters back then just couldn't or didn't talk to each other. For example, Alice had contact with almost everyone except Sabrina. Alice also had bad communication with Makah. She talked to most everyone and always knew what was going on. Luckily, I could talk to almost my whole system. I had good contact with Lucy, Alice, and Clive, while having bad contact with Makah and Brianna, and talking to Sabrina wasn't an option. The others could talk to a lot few alters, like two or three of the seven.

*

MATTHEW SANCHEZ
Matthew was diagnosed with 8
personalities in 2015 at age 16

My alters talk to each other constantly. Santiago keeps himself distant and is in charge of everything that goes on. Occasionally there is conflict, but we usually get things settled without too much strife. Nowadays we have control over switching most of the time.

*

FLOSS SCOTT
Floss was diagnosed with at least
4 personalities in 2016 at age 48

I suffer with other illnesses which are debilitating, and one of my illnesses is non-epileptic seizures, which most of you would have heard of. Now, when I come out of a seizure I am a little girl. Now there are two of them, one is age five and the other age twelve. The alters come when I'm feeling vulnerable, like after a seizure, so one of these is the one who comes out of the seizure. Normally I will conk out shortly after but when I conk out, it's not sleeping, it's more like being in a coma. I have no memory of this, and we don't know which one of me is going to appear after the seizure. I have someone with me at all times and they have to get me home straightaway because I become upset, feel vulnerable and become aggressive. So home and bed is the best place for me.

Each of my alters switch without having conflict with each other. Although I may have no memory of when they switch, at times I still have some control over two of them out of the six or seven. As I'm thinking about all this, I'm finding that I may have more alters than I've noted at the beginning of my story.

*

PAULA SUNDWALL
Paula was diagnosed with dissociative amnesia in 2006 at age
36 and diagnosed with at least 4 personalities in 2014 at age 44

My alters and I don't communicate with each other intentionally at all. I glean things from what other people tell me about their experiences with my alters, and I have some notes and posts that contain information that leads me to believe that my other personalities know each other very well.

My protector as well as my enemy, Jordan, works to keep an adolescent girl in check. If let loose, she cuts me, wrecks cars, and claims to be trying to kill me and us. She is about twelve and is not just self-destructive, but also cold and calculating. She will seize any opportunity to hurt us as quickly as she can. Obviously I have little to no control over any of it, but I have a theory about why they stay inside a lot of the time and don't communicate with me.

I began having severe panic attacks at fifteen. My fear was that I was going crazy and that I would disappear somewhere inside my own mind never to be seen again. I now believe that these attacks were precipitated by an alter coming out, and that would trigger the attack for me. It makes sense to me. People always asked me what triggered my panic attacks, and I said that I had no triggers because they happened randomly, but I believe now that they happened to prevent alters from surfacing.

I found a way to control my panic attacks about two years before my dissociative amnesia diagnosis, which took place in about 2008. I just said something out loud to myself once when one was starting, and I've never had a full-blown panic attack since. It seems silly as I write it down now, but I said, "Some people take drugs to feel this weird. And they do it on purpose!"

I realize this is no great breakthrough for most, but for me the act of hearing it verbally helped convince me that I didn't need to let the panic attack win, and it never did again. But having panic attacks to prevent alters from emerging created a massive barrier between my alters and myself. I had no idea that communication with them, much less making universal rules or guidelines for everyone, was even a remote possibility until I recent went online and started talking to other people with the disorder.

I don't want to get rid of my alters, I just want to get rid of the chaos. I hope to find a way to gain their trust and to mend the burned bridges with them eventually, so we can live together peacefully. I don't have to remain in the court system forever and not be able to drive or go anywhere alone.

*

KERRYJANE VOTH
Kerryjane was diagnosed with
35 alters in 2013 at age 53

Some of my alters know each other. There are groups of alters who only know about themselves and don't communicate outside their groups. There are alters who don't know about the outside world at all. Other alters are aware only of themselves. Some don't like others and will attack them if given a chance. It's really like having a large group composed of different people all living in one place. Like a little village.

*

Scattered
BY SUNSHINE

Sometimes I feel so empty inside, afraid that I may lose control
breaking into a thousand razor sharp pieces,
cutting down through to my soul;
left to bleed internally as my external remains the same
familiar to you as I always was
just now there are different names.

Some you may already have recognized,
while the others will never speak.
Some seem so very angry,
some very timid and weak.
The I gets so tired of everyone playing the fool
while Me is stuck with everyday life
the liars, cheaters, the cruel.

Life is much too complicated as I must hide away
only to speak when spoken to
but never will they hear what I say.
I go about my routine, always trying to keep the peace
while my own internal demons crying out
never again to cease.

Sometimes I feel so empty inside,
afraid that I've lost all control
and the thousand bleeding pieces,
cutting and leaving scars upon my soul.

*

CHAPTER FIVE

Waking Up Someplace Else

I had crossed the line. I was free; but there was no one to welcome me to the land of freedom. I was a stranger in a strange land. -HARRIET TUBMAN

Living with multiple personalities means that different parts have to share one physical body. When an alter or part who is fronting wants to go somewhere, the whole system travels with it, whether they want to or not. When an alter takes the body to an unfamiliar place, maybe even far away, and then retreats within, someone else has to take over. If they aren't familiar with the location, chaos can ensue. Have you ever found yourself in a strange place, and if so, how do you cope?

*

ADRIANNE ALLEN-LANG
Adrianne was diagnosed with 10
personalities in 2015 at age 18

I haven't awakened in strange places. But we're co-conscious with one another. Those who aren't co-conscious don't really front.

*

GAIL BUSWELL
Gail was diagnosed with 13
personalities in 2002 at age 24

I went through a stage of finding myself in the garden at night, often naked. I am not co-conscious with most of my alters, and Sweet Pea, who is eight, just loves being outside. I have now written memos all over my house reminding my others that clothes need to be worn when going outside. I also have a written agreement with Sweet Pea that she must check the weather. If it is cold or wet, she is not allowed outside at night.

*

KATT HART
Katt was diagnosed with hundreds
of personalities in 2011 at age 20

We often come out in different places, and we're rarely on our own because this happens so much. The person or people we're with can then fill us in on what happened while we were missing time, which greatly reduces the panic. There have been some scarier times where we come back after another alter was hurting us, usually sexually. We sometimes have flashbacks or very negative feelings afterward and have to use self-care to calm down and cope until it passes. Things that a lot of us will use to keep calm and distracted are making art, cleaning, cooking, and watching kids shows or movies on television.

*

AMELIA JOUBERT
Amelia was diagnosed with 12
personalities in 2013 at age 15

I do lose time, and often. I don't even realize it happened until later. Sometimes I will think it's a different day of the week than it is, like if it's Tuesday sometimes I think it's Monday, because I don't remember having a Monday. Also, sometimes people will tell me I did something I don't remember doing. Like yesterday I told a friend I was going to see a movie with my mom and she said, "You're going to see that movie again?" Apparently I had already seen it with her, but I have no memory of it. If an alter reads a book or watches a movie and I am not paying attention from the inside, I won't know what happened in that book or movie. I also sometimes will come out in the middle of a conversation, and that can be very confusing.

*

AMANDA LINEBACK
Amanda was diagnosed with hundreds
of personalities in 2013 at age 31

When I first learned I had DID, my system was kind of in shock. None of us were aware of one another, and we had a lot of trouble putting the pieces of each day together. I still do not understand how my boyfriend, Chad, puts up with us. I asked him to tell me about my adventures in dissociation, because I wasn't really around when all the excitement was happening. I had several incidents when Chad was driving and I decided for whatever reason that I needed to do something different and would exit a moving vehicle. Thankfully he knows when I'm not there, and has become very good at predicting my actions, so he was never driving over ten miles an hour.

I went with Chad to visit someone in the hospital. He barely let me out of his sight after all my shenanigans, but someone told him I needed to use the bathroom. An hour or more later I found myself walking in a horrible neighborhood at night about two miles from the hospital. I had stopped at a liquor store at some point because I was carrying an almost finished twenty-four-ounce alcoholic beverage. I called Chad and he came and picked me up. He had been looking for me the entire time, and was in a panic when he picked me up.

One night when Chad came home from work, he thought I was asleep and so worked on his car outside. He kept hearing little noises and noticed flashes of light coming from the inside of one of his vehicles. I was hiding inside this 1981 Scirocco sending S.O.S. signals to him so he would see me. Another time I reached back to fix my ponytail and my hair was gone. I had chopped it off during a flashback. My hair had been down to the middle of my back, and I had cut it up to my chin. Or I would be driving to therapy and all of a sudden seven-year-old Lily would be thrown to the front and find herself driving. It scared her badly and she quickly had to figure out what to do. She just pulled the car over and walked the rest of the way to therapy. She sat in the therapy office for two hours before it was time for our appointment; she just stayed busy playing with baby dolls.

The most shocking experience of all was when I woke up in Texas. I live in Indiana. One of us had a friend who was a truck driver, and decided to ride along with him while he went to Texas for work.

When I woke up, four days had gone by and I was in Texas near the Mexican border with a person I didn't know. Chad thought I was in Louisville at some kind of convention. I thought I was sleeping. We were both mistaken.

We have made several safety contracts that everyone can mutually agree to and sign. This works really well for our system and keeps us all accountable and safe.

*

JANE MACDONALD
Jane was diagnosed with 3 personalities in
2014 at age 35, and currently has 6 alters

Waking up in a strange or unfamiliar place has always been, and continues to be, one of my greatest fears of living with DID. It has happened on numerous occasions. As a result, I tend to isolate myself in my apartment. My largest fear is waking in a place that is not safe, where I may be in physical danger. This has happened once in the past. I woke to find myself standing in the middle of a street with cars honking at me—they had a green light, and I was blocking their path. I have no recollection of where I was before, how long I had been standing in the middle of the street, or why. That was probably one of the most terrifying times when I have woken up because I could have been in real physical danger.

I tend to remain inside my apartment most of the time. However, certain circumstances require me to leave to attend medical appointments, to go to work occasionally, or to run errands. Leaving my apartment always leads to great anxiety and fear that another personality will take over and that I will have no control over what they say or do. I have been fortunate in that many times when I switched, it occurred in safe environments like my doctor or psychiatrist's offices. Although this is scary, I am relatively safe in these circumstances and know that no harm will come to me.

My psychiatrist, in particular, is very good at figuring out who has come out, and is very good at dealing with my younger alters, including the one who is mute and does not speak. More troubling are the times when I switch in public places, such as grocery stores, on public transit, or even just walking down the middle of the street. I have frequently come to in the middle of a grocery store with a cart full of items that I normally wouldn't buy such as candy, ice cream, and other treats. While I am in less physical danger in this situation, it is still upsetting to not know how you got somewhere or for how long you were there. Often when I wake up, I am disoriented and it takes me a while to figure out where I am and to get my bearings. This results in people whispering to one another while staring at me with angry or confused expressions. This doesn't exactly help ease my social anxiety.

Unfortunately, I have not been able to come up with many strategies to deal with these things when they occur. For the most part I try to isolate and stay in my apartment. I am too afraid of someone else being out when I am in public and having no control or awareness of what is going on, what I say, or what I do. I fear someone calling the police and my being taken to a psych ward at a local hospital. I fear others laughing at me, ridiculing me, or even fearing me. I know that isolation is not the answer. There must be some practical solutions to this problem, and I simply have yet to discover any that work.

I can prepare for my littlest ones coming out in medical appointments, for instance, by bringing their favorite teddy bears, blankets or other things that comfort them. However, I can't always do this for them if I am on a public bus or in a grocery store. Then I am helpless, or so it feels that way. I am told that communication is key. Other people with DID have learned to communicate and work with their alters on who will come out and when. Unfortunately, I have never been able to accomplish this with my personalities, although one day I hope this will happen and I will be able to leave my apartment without being paralyzed by the fear and uncertainty of what might happen.

*

CRYSTALIE MATULEWICZ
Crystalie was diagnosed with dissociative
identity disorder in 2015 at age 29

My previous living situation was severely controlled, so I didn't have the actual ability to end up in many strange places. I was only allowed to leave home to go to work, and then I was always escorted. There were times when I would be at work and feel like I had just awakened there. In reality, I had been there for hours, working just like I was supposed to. But while I was physically there, I was mentally somewhere else. I felt as if I had been sleepwalking, lost in some kind of prolonged dream. I attributed it to being tired, since at that time I didn't really know what DID or dissociation was. Looking back, now I can understand those instances as times when I had dissociated.

Once I ran away and began a new life in a new city, I noticed myself often getting lost. It was a new experience for me, as I had never been allowed to do anything independently before. That caused a lot of stress, especially on the inside. I didn't feel entirely safe in my new home, and I didn't yet have any safe places on the outside. My parts were confused. There was a lot of chaos, and as a result, a lot of dissociation. Sometimes I would come back and realize I'd been wandering the streets for a few hours. Fortunately, most of the times it happened it was local enough that I could get back home easily using public transportation. I don't drive, which is probably a good thing. While many people see that as a disadvantage, I think it keeps us from being able to get too far away.

During the first couple of months after I moved, I remember feeling compelled to follow trains. My old home was a few blocks away from the train tracks, so the sound of a train was familiar. Even so, I had never had an interest in trains before; I had never even been on a train. A couple of times I found myself waiting by the tracks, not really remembering how I got there. I didn't think much of it, just found it to be slightly annoying. I found out later on that one of my parts was trying to get on a train to return to our former home. I had to explain that we had moved and were never going back to that place. I haven't wandered off to the tracks since.

There were also a few instances in which I found myself in the emergency room of a hospital without remembering actually going there. It was probably better that I ended up there, as they were instances when I had felt extremely unstable prior to going there. It confused the hospital staff, however, when I switched from being suicidal to appearing perfectly fine.

Because I was still new to the area, most places were unfamiliar to me. When I would come back from being dissociated, I wouldn't know where I was, even if it was just a couple of miles away from home. The GPS on my phone became my lifesaver. I made sure to carry a backpack with me at all times, with a phone charger, a card with my address, and a paper with phone numbers to call and instructions in case we got lost or needed help.

Now that I'm more familiar with the area, and more familiar with my parts and my system, these experiences have become less frequent and less troublesome. I encourage my parts to come out in safe places, like at therapy and at home. There are instances when I am triggered by something and dissociate when out somewhere, but I make an effort to ground myself so we don't end up getting lost. Fortunately, we haven't had any major problems.

*

ALICIA PETTIS
Alicia was diagnosed with 40
personalities in 2015 at age 16

I remember coming back in the middle of an alleyway. My hands were bleeding and I had several red marks that would later turn into bruises. It was terrifying to not know where I was, how I got there, or what had happened. My alters used to get confused and scared when they came out in a new environment that was foreign to them. Since my diagnosis, my alters are more open to others. Now they just ask whoever is around them what happened, if another alter hadn't already informed them. As for me, I got better at dealing with new environments and coming back to something that wasn't there before.

*

SUNSHINE PURCELL
Denise was diagnosed with 17
personalities in 1995 at age 30

I've found myself in a Walmart parking lot, driving down a strange road, or going to a store. And every day at least twice I am out, so to speak, for a few minutes to a few hours, and don't know where I am. I don't see or feel anything. It's as though I stepped out of my body. I awake to find I've eaten food I don't like, toys that were played with, a stuffed animal and favorite blanket on the couch, and drawings or notes I haven't written. To minimize what happens is impossible for me right now. That's why I am pretty much stay-at-home mom to the alters I only know by name.

If it's a trigger time, like spring is for the little ones, there is a fear of lilac trees and grandfatherly figures. Sometimes that's impossible to predict. They will cry and panic, have a flashback and terror thoughts. If I am aware of the trigger times for each, I try to make a plan of being safe and only being out for a little while, so as not to cause too much stress. I can feel the triggers coming, peaking, and when they start to leave. It's horrible, because I not only feel my feelings, but I feel their feelings too, which are really mine that I don't feel at that time, along with any feelings the rest have. Maybe one has a similar incident, but not exactly; it can end up a domino effect.

*

ERICKA REEVE
Ericka was diagnosed with over
25 personalities in 2013 at age 26

This has happened many, many, many times, and as far back as I can remember. As I got older it would last for longer periods of time, and the aftermath was usually worse.

I've ended up in apartments I didn't recognize that ended up being my own. My name was on the lease; not always my own signature, but my name nonetheless. I've ended up in hospitals and other places, as well as other states and even another country once. Yep, good old Canada.

How did I cope? Not well. I don't remember much about any of those experiences. They felt like a dream, the small moments I was able to see and experience. Until recently I just chalked most of those occurrences up to a nightmare or night terror, telling myself it couldn't have happened. Unfortunately, I was wrong. Dead wrong.

I remember various smells of some of these instances, some sounds, even tastes. Hospitals and certain medications have a distinct smell and taste. That's what I remember. My parts would take over when I became too overwhelmed, or in situations they didn't believe I could or can't handle. I think they were trying to show me what was wrong, that I was not crazy and that I did not have some rare brain tumor. It sounds bizarre, but that's what I was thinking. I knew I lost time. That was it. I still can't tell you why it had occurred so frequently, or for such lengths of time.

I did not cope well and I still struggle with the blackouts when they take over. My alters take over not because of their own fear, but because of my fear, or the fear they feel from a smaller, younger, or weaker alter. They protect, and do it shockingly well.

*

CHRIS ROBIN
Chris was diagnosed with at least
7 personalities in 2013 at age 49

I often wake up with the sense of not knowing where I am. It's not until I can snap myself out of the sleepy slumber and fully take in my surroundings that I catch my brain up with my body and location. I have had times when I have found something I did during the night that I don't remember doing. I have written notes to myself, found journal writings on my computer, and even woke once to find my bathroom in a mess. In the past, the only way I could try to handle it or cope with it was by pretending it never happened, and hiding it deep in a box and avoiding the sight of that container. I didn't know that I was really dissociating. I'm learning to recognize when it's happening, and trying to learn compassion and understanding about why I do that. Therapy is teaching me how to open some of those boxes and face them, when before I just avoided them.

*

QUINN ROSE
Quinn was diagnosed with 9
personalities in 2016 at age 21

I blacked out while driving and ended up in another state. I didn't know what to do, so I just turned around. I've also awakened in the bed of someone I didn't know. I freaked out and ran away. I try to keep myself surrounded by people who can keep an eye on me so I don't end up in strange places. It's terrifying not knowing.

*

AYA SAKURA
Aya has been living with 7
personalities since childhood

Waking up in strange places happens quite a lot. No matter where I am, the first thing I always do after a blackout is check the date, time, calendar, where I am, and what I am doing. That helps a bit to fill the gaps in my memory, and I might get clues as to what happened and who was out. It also helps me to calm down and ground myself by doing that, because I know how much time I lost.

I have fast switches most of the time. After a sudden switch, one which takes a second, I mostly have absolutely no clue of what's going on and I just fall silent for a second to recollect myself and to decide how I am going to act and react. Most of the time this means I have to improvise, especially when I am in the middle of an action. The first moments (and in extreme cases, hours) after such a switch, I am very sharp on the clues of my surroundings. From those clues I might be able to figure out my location. One time I switched back while Clive was getting us home by train after a college fieldtrip. I woke up in a moving train without knowing the next stop, the destination of the train, or where I should get off. By checking the calendar, date and time, I figured I was probably getting home. After figuring out in which train I was and where this train was headed, I managed to get out at the right stop and get on my next train.

125

When we switch very slowly, for example over the course of a few hours, I mostly have a vague idea of what's going on. In these cases, I'm able to flawlessly continue with whatever it was we were doing, but not if either of my alters was doing something I am not able to do. But I still check the time, date, how much time I lost, and my calendar, and that helps me to fill the gaps.

Slow switches sometimes also mean I get to be co-conscious with my alters. If so, I can talk with them and most of the time they'll talk me through everything, except if I'm not allowed to know for some reason. Like I said, my surroundings tell me a lot about what's going on.

I have a few friends who know about my alters and accept them. It happens sometimes that I switch while around my friends. If I come back then, I just ask them what happened and they'll tell me, or give me a short summary of what happened while I was gone. I only ask my friends, though, when we aren't around any people who know me but don't know of my DID. I don't want people to figure out what's going on with me. When I am around people I know, who don't know about my DID, I stay in the background as much as possible. I just look around a bit to see how the situation develops, how people talk and react to me, and then I adjust my behavior to their expectations, while hoping they don't notice anything.

*

MATTHEW SANCHEZ
Matthew was diagnosed with 8
personalities in 2015 at age 16

About two years ago I woke sitting on a park bench in the rain with my big green coat on. I had an empty candy wrapper and a cracked pair of sunglasses in my pocket. My feet hurt, and my phone had dozens of missed calls and texts from my mother. I wasn't scared, because I was awakened on purpose by Santiago, my protector. Earlier that day he had gotten so upset that he decided to take a walk. He was so upset that he didn't pay attention to where he was going. He got lost in my neighborhood, and angrily trudged around in the rain for hours.

Another incident involved Santiago and my girlfriend. One day he woke up and she was sleeping with her arms wrapped around his waist. He was so uncomfortable that he got up and stayed awake the rest of the night.

My strategy is communication and rules. When I communicate to my alters, they usually listen. Making to-do lists and staying on task is extremely important for us. We help instruct each other and get through each day with as much cooperation as possible.

*

FLOSS SCOTT
Floss was diagnosed with at least
4 personalities in 2016 at age 48

I have awakened feeling like I don't know how I got here, or wondering what I was doing here. It was the scariest feeling ever, and

I fear having to experience that again. Lucky for me, I can't go out without a caregiver and I can't drive anymore either. So this way my caregiver can always explain to me why I may be in a strange place.

*

PAULA SUNDWALL
Paula was diagnosed with dissociative amnesia in 2006 at age
36 and diagnosed with at least 4 personalities in 2014 at age 44

I rarely come to in an unexpected place, but when I do, it's not as terrifying as one might expect, given my many years of blackout drinking, especially in college. Still, coming back to find myself somewhere strange is not a good feeling because I no longer have alcohol to blame it on, and I'm fully accountable for the things I've done while not actually myself.

Twice I've come back to find myself in a hospital. One time I was just about to be admitted to a psych ward because I'd gone to a walk-in clinic and had been unable to fill out the form identifying myself. The other time I awakened in a psych ward after crashing my car into a retaining wall. I told police that my kids were safe at their dad's so it was okay for me to die, and then refused to speak again after that.

I try to take everything in stride and to remain calm. For some reason, the hardest part for me is to read documents describing me doing and saying things I don't remember, such as police reports or doctor's notes. It's like watching a movie of yourself that you have no attachment to. I see me, but I don't feel me.

The biggest problem with coming to, particularly in strange or difficult situations, is having to explain myself. So very few people know or understand anything about DID. I find myself explaining it over and over, and getting the same puzzled or outright disbelieving responses.

*

KERRYJANE VOTH
Kerryjane was diagnosed with
35 alters in 2013 at age 53

I've had that waking-up experience a lot. It still happens to me, but since being in therapy and becoming co-conscious, it happens less now than in the past. It used to trigger into a panic or anxiety attack that would completely debilitate me. Just anticipating the panic or anxiety was bad enough. Not understanding what was happening was just terrifying, and very confusing. I would retreat to my home and not go out, or I would retreat to a single room in my home and not leave it unless I absolutely had to.

Since being in therapy, I've learned what is going on with the executive functioning of my brain during those moments, and have been developing what is called co-consciousness, which is creating the awareness that helps to lessen these episodes of lost time and memory. Now when it happens, I say to myself, "Oh, look at that. We are waking up because we have not been co-conscious, and we have just switched into another alter. How interesting is that?" And then I go on with my day.

I have learned through therapy that staying curious trumps fear every single time.

*

*

Artwork by Andre
Denise Purcell's alter
www.sisterdiarieswithsunshine.com

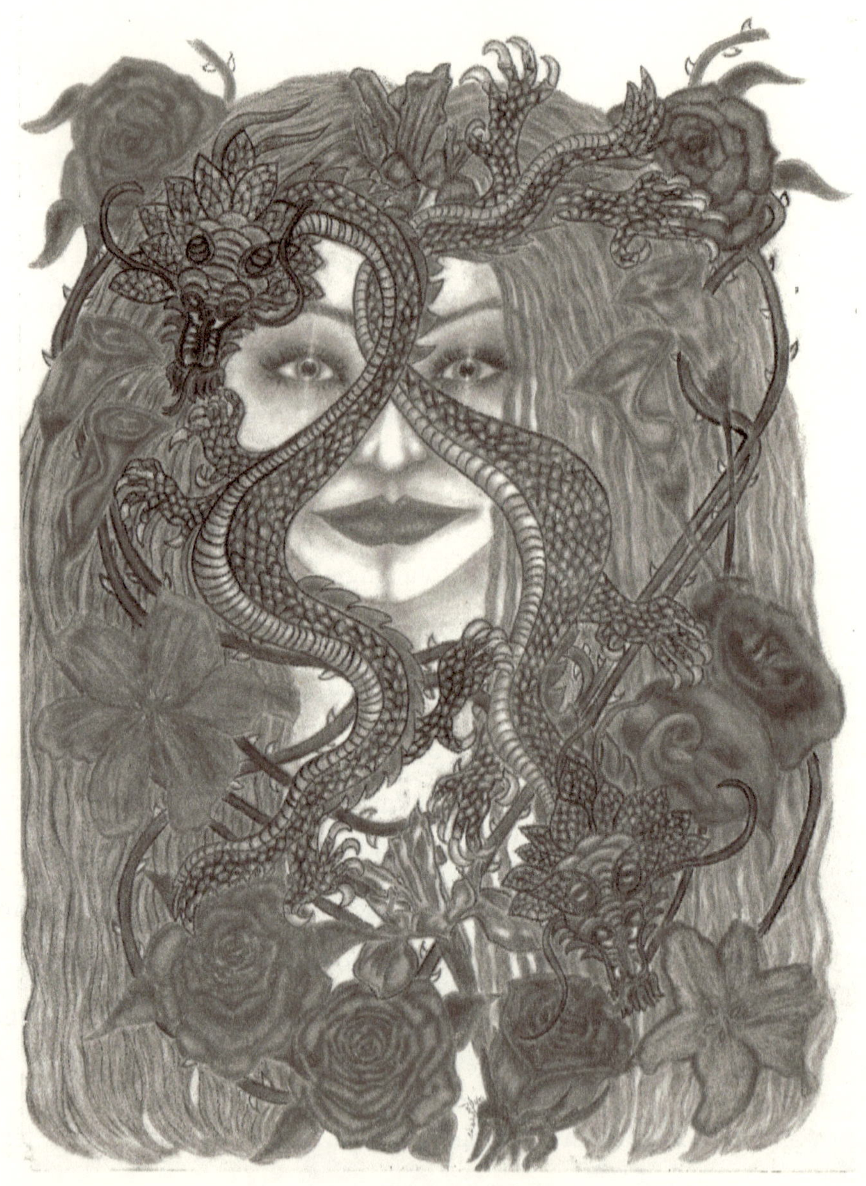

CHAPTER SIX

Our Daily Routine

So, to come In with a set routine is something I've never believed in. It should depend on how you feel, because you play what you feel. -BUDDY RICH

Most people have a daily routine of some sort. For some, that includes a career or school, and for others it includes children. Do your different personalities allow you to work or attend school? Are those around you aware of your alters?

*

ADRIANNE ALLEN-LANG
Adrianne was diagnosed with 10
personalities in 2015 at age 18

I'm studying grade eleven at the moment. My teachers and the school board are aware of my DID, but my classmates are not. We all just pretend to be me if I'm not fronting. We've got a routine where the others try not to come out unless needed during class. Breaks between classes are their times to add to or finish any work, and after I finish homework and my son goes to bed, then they get to come out and do their own thing and finish the day's chores.

*

GAIL BUSWELL
Gail was diagnosed with 13
personalities in 2002 at age 24

I am unable to work due to not being co-conscious of my others. I have no idea how we manage to run a home. We just do.

*

KATT HART
Katt was diagnosed with hundreds
of personalities in 2011 at age 20

Unfortunately, we aren't able to work, because we're still unable to control switching and still have very strong reactions to triggers that come up often in daily life. At home we struggle to keep on top of housework and cooking, because of having chronic pain. There are some alters who manage the pain very well or can't feel it, and they can do a lot of housework because of it. We rely very much on those alters. Unfortunately, they can't always come out to keep on top of things, but they do as often as they can and it's a great help!

One of the difficult parts of keeping up with a routine at home is that some alters are children who can't actually do things like cook or clean. When they're out we usually end up with a big mess of toys, and they'll eat cereal or candy all day which means we also come back to feeling quite sick.

*
AMELIA JOUBERT
Amelia was diagnosed with 12
personalities in 2013 at age 15

I just started college and I enjoy it. We haven't really gotten into the full swing of things, but we had a few things in high school that helped us. One thing we did was find who was good at what. Scarlet is best at math, so she took those classes. Ahina is good at science. Jax is good at reading comprehension, and I (Amelia) am a good writer, so we share English subjects. We also have very good communication, so we can talk to each other during a test and answer questions together. We sometimes study together too. Communication used to be a mess, but now runs more smoothly.

*
AMANDA LINEBACK
Amanda was diagnosed with hundreds
of personalities in 2013 at age 31

I am currently on disability because of my mental health. Along with my DID, I also have obsessive-compulsive disorder, attention deficit hyperactivity disorder, complex posttraumatic stress disorder, panic disorder with agoraphobia, and major depressive disorder. I worked and went to school without any problems for the majority of my life. I was a pre-med major and was a National Collegiate Honors Scholar with two children under the age of four. I went from being able to take on the world to not even being able to leave my house. I have come a long way and I rejoice in the little victories. I am proud of where I am and how hard we have worked to get here. I am to the point where if this is as stable and functional as I can get, I will be happy with that. I never thought I would be able to be alone or have any kind of normality again. I write in a journal, and when I feel discouraged I look at my old entries to remind myself that I am doing all the things I thought I would never be able to do again.

*

JANE MACDONALD
Jane was diagnosed with 3 personalities in
2014 at age 35, and currently has 6 alters

Since I have been diagnosed with DID I have been largely unable to work or attend school. I currently have a part-time job, but work only one day a month. Even that can be challenging, and I have had days when I was not able to attend, or when I did attend but was completely unable to work.

I consider myself fortunate in that my employer is actually a friend of mine and so I felt comfortable telling her about my diagnosis. Unfortunately, she doesn't always understand what it means to have other personalities or alters come out. She tends to think of DID as a personality disorder, largely because of its former name. She does know when I am showing signs of one of my alters being out, and is very understanding and helpful with my little ones in particular. She has learned that if my youngest one comes out, it is best to give her simple tasks to do like a puzzle or drawing, or if she is able, to have her do the dishes and cleaning. It keeps my alter distracted. It also serves to prevent unnecessary conversations with coworkers who are, by and large, unaware of my DID with the exception of one individual.

There is, however, always a fear that an alter will come out at work who is more aggressive or destructive, that he or she will say or do something to upset or harm others. I've had coworkers comment "You didn't seem yourself last week," and I don't always know what to say. I usually dismiss it as being particularly tired or having some stressful situation going on. Most of the time they seem to accept this explanation, but I'm extremely self-conscious about revealing that I have other personalities. I fear the reaction of coworkers and others who may not understand what DID is about, who may think I am faking it or doing it for the attention.

I am always nervous about losing time, losing control, and even losing my friends. I am confident that I would not lose my current job because of my DID, but at the same time I do have a history of losing previous jobs for this very reason. The difference with these other jobs was that I wasn't aware of my DID at the time, didn't understand what was going on, and was too afraid to mention anything to my employers. As a result, other personalities would emerge and say or do things that were incorrect or inappropriate, and I would lose the job. I look forward to a day when all employers are more understanding and open to accommodating people with DID, or any mental illness, but I fear that day is a long way off. In the meantime, we do the best we can.

School was a different matter. When I was in school I had the symptoms of DID but not the diagnosis. This made functioning incredibly difficult. If an alter came out in class, I couldn't control what he or she said or did. I was rarely co-conscious, although this has improved recently, and so I would often have no memory of what was said in a particular lecture. It was extremely difficult to take tests, because sometimes one of my other alters would come out and not know how to answer the questions. Imagine the challenges of having a two-year-old alter come out during the middle of a fourth-year university statistics course! I was fortunate to have notetakers for many of my classes (for learning disability reasons, not because of my DID) as well as tutors. I credit these individuals with enabling me to complete my university degree. Frankly, without their assistance I would not have stood a chance.

Unfortunately, I was unable to complete my college program because it involved doing a field placement in a social service agency, and no support was offered or available to people with mental health disabilities. You were expected to work full-time, often thirty to forty hours a week. There was simply no way that I would have been able to cope with those kinds of demands, especially in a professional setting with no support in place should an alter come out. I often think of returning and trying to finish my program, but I don't feel I can do this until I gain more of an under-standing of my alters, and a greater capacity to control what alters are out at any given time, and greater confidence in how to handle it when a personality comes out in a field placement situation.

Routines at home are also an ongoing concern. I, myself, struggle to find the motivation or energy to complete the basic tasks of cooking, cleaning, organizing, etc. My personalities, particularly my youngest ones, do not take on any such responsibilities. Only one alter, a teenage one, tends to do bouts of cleaning, only, I believe, because she is restless and can't sit still. Either way, I am glad and grateful for the help! However, often there are times when I will go weeks or months without doing a thorough cleaning, only doing the very basics such as washing enough dishes to eat off of, or washing enough clothes so I have something to wear for a few days. While this is not entirely because of my DID, having other personalities who refuse to take on household tasks doesn't make the situation any easier.

*

CRYSTALIE MATULEWICZ
Crystalie was diagnosed with dissociative
identity disorder in 2015 at age 29

I got a new job just weeks after running away from home, and I have been able to keep that same job for over a year now. It is only part-time, as that is about as much as I can handle. I also go to school and go to therapy a couple of times a week, and working full time would be too much stress.

I work in retail, which anyone who has ever worked in retail knows is not an easy job. There's a lot of expectations, deadlines, social interactions, and many times a high amount of stress. That can be difficult for any singleton to handle. When you're a multiple with DID, it can make things especially complicated.

When I am under an excessive amount of stress, I dissociate. When it gets to that point, I rarely have control over it. There have been instances at work when I have dissociated. Usually it's just for a couple of hours and then I come back to the front, with a huge headache and a lot of confusion. The first few times it happened, I tried not to acknowledge that it happened at all. A couple of people would ask if I was okay, that I seemed out of it, and I would just say I wasn't feeling well. There's no easy way to explain what was really going on.

I knew it was important to stay grounded at work so I could do what was needed, but I quickly realized it wouldn't work out that way all the time. Sometimes a coworker would point out how my choice would change, and I would play it off. I got frustrated with my coworker one time because I insisted the work wasn't mine, only to realize that I was the only person (in body) who did that job. I couldn't recognize the handwriting on my paperwork because it was another part's handwriting. I needed to at least know that we could still do the job even when I was out of it. Most times we've been able to get the work done. I'd occasionally have a part come out that would have no idea what he or she was doing. It caused a lot of embarrassment at work when someone asked what happened and I couldn't remember, but fortunately it has never been anything too detrimental.

I did make the decision to come forward to my coworkers about some of my mental health struggles. I knew that none of them had any background in mental health, so going full DID would be like explaining calculus to a kindergartner. I started out disclosing my PTSD, and my coworkers were supportive and receptive to learning more. So little by little I built up to disclosing about my dissociative issues. It was helpful for me, because I needed them to understand why it was important for me not to get so stressed out, and I needed them to know how they could help me. I also didn't want them to be confused as to why I acted differently all of a sudden. I worried that management would think I was under the influence, when in reality I was just under the influence of another alter. It is much easier at work now, and I don't feel like I have to hide who I am.

I briefly worked another retail job at a well-known baby store, but had to quit after less than a week. The store environment ended up being a constant trigger for me. I saw happy families, mothers who were loving and nurturing their infant children—the love that I never got to experience from my own parents. Some of my parts didn't understand why we didn't have a mother who loved us. They cried. I cried. It was too painful, and I was still grieving my own losses, so I ended up leaving.

In addition to working, I also attend graduate school. Most of the coursework is online, so it is much easier to get my work done when I can. I was in graduate school before, but I had to drop out. It wasn't for lack of trying. In fact, I did really well in the program. I had a 4.0 GPA, received high regards from my professors, and even scored above the national average on the CPCE. I was so proud of myself and my system for doing so well. And then I got a notice that someone had anonymously reported me to the head of the department for having DID and other mental health issues, which they found out by finding my online blog. All of a sudden the great work I did, and was still doing, didn't matter. My diagnosis was a concern. The school said I was a perceived threat and safety risk to others. I didn't feel like I was being treated fairly, so I left.

My parts know that school things are important and need to get done on a schedule. Some of my younger parts are, not surprisingly, bored with schoolwork. I am actually the one most interested in academic work, so I handle the school-related things myself. It makes it easier for all of us, and no one has to do anything they don't want to do.

*

ALICIA PETTIS
Alicia was diagnosed with 40
personalities in 2015 at age 16

Attending school is about as challenging as hiding my DID when I was younger. My alters try to help me out with schooling by taking notes for me or writing down my assignments, but they never write it down where I can find it. For hours I'm left searching for an assignment that should take about five minutes. My teachers are nice about it and understand that sometimes it's not Alicia who is attending class. They normally try to help out as much as possible. While my teachers are one hundred percent aware, my classmates are not. Except for my friends who are understanding and know all of my alters, my classmates have no clue. It becomes a long discussion when an alter is out, and they don't understand why teachers and friends are calling them one name when they believe my name is something else. Besides that, my alters do what they have to if they're out. They might protest, but they will help.

*

SUNSHINE PURCELL
Denise was diagnosed with 17
personalities in 1995 at age 30

I worked for years before it became unbearable. I have been on disability since. None of my coworkers ever found out. My family knew something was wrong, but until I had a diagnosis, they didn't know. As far as routines go, I am the main person who is out. I do most of the daily chores. If there needs to be interaction with people like doctor appointments, the Smart One comes out and makes sure everything is addressed. I have told my primary care provider and specialists about my DID just in case one alter comes out during a visit. Things like gynecologists have to be taken with caution, and women physicians. Entertaining people around holidays is The Mother's job. The male alters do things like bring in wood. It's really a crapshoot when it comes to day-to-day life. If given instructions or specific duties like writing this, it's about not letting people down. If we let anyone down, they take their love or friendship away.

*

ERICKA REEVE
Ericka was diagnosed with over 25
personalities in 2013 at age 26

This is another tricky question for me. When I was in high school, it was an ongoing joke amongst people who were closer to me that I had multiple personalities. Funny, yet not so funny now. I went to a couple of colleges but couldn't handle being around people. I still don't remember most of it. I can't tell you the years I attended or classmates, and only vaguely remember one of my professors. I was still unaware at that point, and couldn't handle it. No one in any job or academic institution was ever aware that I am plural. And you wouldn't know unless we wanted you to. It kind of defeats the purpose for us to protect her IF we make it clear that we're there . . . duh.

As for home, I am barely able to function. Some days are better than others, and therapy is greatly helping. It took over a decade, but with the persistence of one particular part we found a great therapist. Minny typically will do housework and cooking, grocery shopping, and things like that. She as well as some younger parts help me with the pets. Some really enjoy playing with our ferrets. We rescue and foster them, and it gives my life some semblance of purpose and normality. They're very affectionate and, on harder days, they really are fantastic.

*

CHRIS ROBIN
Chris was diagnosed with at least
7 personalities in 2013 at age 49

I was able to go through college and work as a teacher for thirty years. In fact, I think I am a hard worker, and work has given me the strongest ability to compartmentalize. Work has become my safest coping device. I am able to put all the parts of me in safe environments and somehow almost always keep them from interfering with my work. I do value the structure and consistency of work. It helps to be surrounded by coworkers who understand my quirks, value my opinions, and work with me to create an environment that provides structure, schedule and pattern. I don't think any of my coworkers know that I have DID, or at least have never shown or told me they suspected anything like that. But I know that since the death of my partner of twenty-five years the uneasiness of life has changed all of me, and they do notice those changes.

Since my DID diagnosis, I am much more aware of when parts of me interfere or enter my work environment. I suspect that they have always done that, but it is much harder now to keep them at bay or out of sight. Fortunately, I retired from teaching and I don't have to spend so much mental, emotional and cognitive energy every day keeping my parts in their place, and I might be able to learn better, healthier coping skills. Going to therapy regularly is helping with that. I am learning to ask for help and build a toolbox of coping skills to use when parts of me become more active. I never realized that hiding them away only made them feel less valued and caused more distress.

*

QUINN ROSE
Quinn was diagnosed with 9
personalities in 2016 at age 21

I do work. I actually own my own company now. I think my alters only come out when I am triggered, though lately it's been quite frequent due to dealing with so much physical pain. We just try to manage to be as unnoticeable as possible.

*

AYA SAKURA
Aya has been living with 7
personalities since childhood

My DID allows me to attend school. I finished high school with very good results (thank you, Lucy), and am now attending University of Applied Sciences. I am currently studying human resource management and am in my second year. I was also able to do a six-week internship in my first year.

High school in the Netherlands is divided in two parts. The first three years you take almost all the subjects the school provides, and for the last two years the student chooses a specialization. Halfway through high school I chose mathematics, physics, chemistry, biology, and computer sciences as my specialization subjects, and my standard courses were English, Dutch (my native language), sociology, physical education, and cultural and artistic education. While in high school I had seven personalities including myself, and some of them helped me through some of the high school subjects.

I will mostly be talking about my last two years, as I know most of those years in terms of who was around then, and what the load balancing was. Alice had always been fluent in English; she did not speak Dutch, even if we tried to teach her. At the start of my third year, after one teacher had been "really mean" according to Alice, she began taking my English lessons and tests. Later, in my fourth and fifth year, Brianna also began taking English, as it interested her. I picked up English through speaking with my alters in English, reading, and the internet.

I always hated physical education and was really bad at it, so from the beginning of high school to the end of it, Alice took my P.E. classes. Alice didn't have to speak, so that was no problem at all and she absolutely loved those classes, as she was a very active girl. I had no problem with biology, Dutch, sociology, and cultural and artistic education, so I did those myself. I sometimes had a bit of trouble with Dutch, so Makah, who was very smart and a native Dutch speaker, helped me out with that every once in a while. Math was a subject I really liked and enjoyed, but I found it quite difficult. Lucy was very smart, and in my first three years she helped me with that. During the last two years Clive took my math with the support of Lucy, as he has taken an interest in economics and math.

Since I could not really handle physics and chemistry, though I really did like the practical side of them, Lucy was in charge of these two subjects. Computer sciences was mostly Alice's job. She was very good with computers, but couldn't speak or understand Dutch, so I was the one who talked with the group and told her what to do. This was possible since me and my group members were almost always working by ourselves without much communication. The program we had to work in was in English, so as soon as we were allowed to use the computer, Alice would take over. This was sometimes very complicated because of the homework. I did the sports and gave swimming lessons with a limited amount of time, so Makah took it upon herself to plan everything and make sure everyone got everything done on time. Sabrina helped with that. They both talked to different alters, since not everyone had contact with everyone. Sayu took this job halfway through my fourth year, when Makah and Sabrina merged (they became Sayu together). Sayu did this for a year and then Lucy took the job just before my high school final exams after Sayu disappeared—either merged or hiding, I'm not sure which.

After I finished high school, I enrolled in a Bachelor's of biology and medical laboratory research. I broke this course off after three months, after someone thought I was unfit for this specific course and dangerous in a lab. I worked for a year as a cashier and mail delivery girl. This worked out pretty well, since at this point only two alters and me were active. Everyone else had gone into hiding or merged because of the shock caused by the sudden stop of my bachelor's program. Both my alters knew the mail delivery route, and they would take responsibility and deliver the mail if needed. They also quietly learned how to do cashier work, but they left that for me most of the time.

Last year I started another degree program in human resource management. I have a lot of free time, and Brianna and Clive always take notes for me when they are out in class. I have an electronic agenda which always gives reminders for classes and deadlines. Instead of having a separate notebook for each class, I have one so that it's easy to for my alters to pack my bag for class. I also have a notebook in which we write homework and messages to each other, so that we know what's going on. This works really well for us, and I managed to advance to my second year. We also have a rule that school time is my time, so I miss as few lessons as possible. Having attendance also really helped. While I had my internship, I had to work from 8 a.m. to 5 p.m.

My alters did not come out during these hours, as I made it clear this internship was very important for me. When I had difficult moments, they became co-conscious to help me. Most of the time Brianna woke up and brought me to work and Clive brought me back home.

*

MATTHEW SANCHEZ
Matthew was diagnosed with 8
personalities in 2015 at age 16

My DID was a punch to my academic career. I was a straight-A student until my alters began goofing around and acting out during school. I missed so many days that I had to retake my classes. My classmates and teachers were never aware, they just thought I was a bad kid. Now, school and work are extremely manageable. Some of my alters have excellent recall and help me in all parts of school. Two or more heads is definitely better than one.

*

FLOSS SCOTT
Floss was diagnosed with at least
4 personalities in 2016 at age 48

One of my strongest alters is the one who is organized, never misses an appointment, is always on time, etc. She's a perfectionist and becomes vicious if anyone stops her from being on time. She hates a mess, too. I suffer from seizures too, and alters would switch by the time I came around. This, along with my DID, caused my problems at school and college. From aged twelve to sixteen, I didn't manage well the first couple of years at secondary school. I hardly attended after the first few months. I think I was dropped down a set, and that upset me so one of my negative alters came out who hated school. Once I was in year nine, I missed only one or two days over the last three years of secondary school.

The teacher would explain the work we had to do, but it was like I wasn't there so she would have to explain three or four times before I could comprehend. Even then, I would still go back to ask more questions. I was easily distracted but produced extremely good work when focused. I was excellent at practical work, whether I had done it before or not. I found it remarkable that I can do things I've never done before. I've produced superb things, especially cooking, baking, sewing, crafts, painting, decorating, and artwork. My brain could process some stuff like a computer and just download all the contents. I've never been able to work that one out.

On the downside, I got bored very easily and wouldn't finish long projects. Instead, I would start something else that was interesting. This was only if something became boring, though.

I was a very active child and adult, and find it difficult to sit still and focus. Over the years I have tried to train myself to focus more, but still have problems. I also had problems with looking at words. I would read a book from the back to the beginning. I never liked reading even though I was okay at it, although I still find it difficult to pronounce big words. Also, sometimes when I look at words, the letters seem all jumbled up, and I see words that are not there. So now I have one of the children read my mail and help manage my appointments, etc.

*

PAULA SUNDWALL
Paula was diagnosed with dissociative amnesia in 2006 at age
36 and diagnosed with at least 4 personalities in 2014 at age 44

Since my initial diagnosis about seven years ago, I've had six jobs. The DID interferes with everything and makes it hard to be reliable. I don't know how or why it seemed to be dormant for so long, but I used to have a completely normal life (minus the binge drinking). I finished college and even went back several years ago to get my master's in psychology.

I was married with two children, and had a successful career. But my marriage was an unhappy one, and when I got divorced that's when my life really started to unravel. My parents took my ex-husband's side, because he told them lies about me and they believed him. I think having my entire family turn on me may have been a trigger of some kind.

My career began to crumble as the real estate market began to dive in 2007 and 2008. Emotionally, financially, romantically, my whole life was falling apart piece by piece. It was just one trauma after another for about seven years, until finally I had a breakdown and was diagnosed as bipolar.

In college, I had been diagnosed with borderline personality disorder. This is a common diagnosis for people with DID. After the bipolar diagnosis I finally quit drinking, but that's when the dissociative episodes started. Since then, my life has continued to spiral. I went from owning multiple properties and living a very nice life with my children to renting a room in a house and having my parents (who are back in my life now, fifteen years later) drive me to all my appointments and keep track like I'm a child.

I now have very little freedom, no money of my own, and very few friends. The ones who weren't scared by my problems mostly ended up being the type who saw my disability as an opportunity to take advantage of me, and so I've had to weed them down to almost none.

Luckily, both my sons are grown now, and I'm very open with them about my experiences. They are such smart, loving children who don't treat me any differently. Now that they're grown, they have lives of their own so I don't get to see them nearly as often as I'd like. I try not to let my drastic lifestyle changes get me too down. I'm an optimistic person and I'd like to think that something good will come from all this. I'm a very spiritual person and believe God has a plan for me, so I try to look at everything as learning experiences instead of just horrible setbacks.

*

KERRYJANE VOTH
Kerryjane was diagnosed with
35 alters in 2013 at age 53

DID has totally interfered with my ability to be employed. Before being diagnosed, I was able to function better if I was in an environment that allowed for a more entrepreneurial experience. I learned this the hard way through having to leave one job after another. Eventually I was able to run my own sport fishing business. I never felt comfortable working in a team environment, because I have a hard time trusting people's intentions. I have a hard time remembering conversations, commitments, times, and dates, so I've been vulnerable to being manipulated or controlled.

Since being in therapy, it has become apparent that my system is so vast—over thirty-five alters—that it's a full-time job in and of itself to manage all the alters on a daily basis, which has now made working impossible. I've been working on creating communication between alters, and asking for better cooperation. I hold board meetings, and call everyone in to listen and give their input. I ask for suggestions and ideas to help solve problems, and I encourage and facilitate well suited alters to pair or group up to tackle certain problems. All of this has to be delivered with an open, curious, and respectful attitude. If there are any disputes or negative responses, these must be addressed first before proceeding. In other words, we have to go through a process that will bring us all to an agreement before we can move forward with things in the outside world, even with the simplest of tasks like sleeping, eating, personal hygiene, cooking, shopping, budgeting, socializing, etc. Because without group consensus, the body will either not respond or else shut down completely by switching into a sleep alter. It is the ultimate example of working democracy. This is time consuming and energy consuming to the body, and many days the body will be totally exhausted and need extra daytime naps. I'm now on disability.

*

Voices
BY SUNSHINE

Stumbling through life's mazes, obstacles at every turn,
finding the way to freedom, is all I ever yearn.

When life gets too hard, a continual rainy day,
I curl up like a ball and shut myself away,
looking out from inside myself and feeling all alone,
never finding the words to describe, what comes is just a moan.

Did I or didn't I, are questions frequently I ask,
what person have I become who hides behind my mask?
When does it stop, the voices in my head?
"Of course I did not tell you," forget what I've just said.

The walls built to protect have become bars to hold me tight,
and the very thing I'm looking for seems so very out of sight.
I have friends who play the game of "knowing how I feel,"
but what they do not realize is who they see may not be real.

I'm consciously aware of how unconscious I may seem,
that reality somehow exists between the present and in my dream.
Unfamiliar faces patiently awaiting, watching me,
for in my moment of weakness, they'll act and be set free
to do what they will, and say what they must,
leaving a trail of denial, powerless feelings of distrust,

They say it's a gift, a mind's protection at any cost,
but they have never felt the feelings, mostly I just feel lost,
looking out and seeing people able to do what they may,
while I sit and wonder, what do their voices say?
The best hope for me is for no more fighting within my head,
but the biggest fear of all is
if the voices all went dead.

*

CHAPTER SEVEN

Going Out in Public

Life is like playing a violin solo in public and learning
the instrument as one goes on. -SAMUEL BUTLER

Dissociative identity disorder requires an arrangement or agreement among the alters when going out in public, especially with the young alters, to prevent uncomfortable situations. What strategies do you agree upon to manage when out in public? Do you fear alters breaking this agreement in public?

*

ADRIANNE ALLEN-LANG
Adrianne was diagnosed with 10
personalities in 2015 at age 18

This is not a fear of mine.

*

GAIL BUSWELL
Gail was diagnosed with 13
personalities in 2002 at age 24

I very rarely go out in public. When I do, it is very well planned out so all my others know exactly where we are going and why. I try to stay present as much as possible to avoid embarrassment. If my head is foggy, which happens a lot, I refuse to leave the house.

*

KATT HART
Katt was diagnosed with hundreds
of personalities in 2011 at age 20

We don't often go out alone because of this disagreement. We've been known to go shopping and stand in the same aisle for a long time, staring at the same section and making noises or mumbling to ourselves because different alters have different ideas on what's wanted or needed. When our partner or friends are with us, they help us come to decisions easier or else ask some of the alters to step back so a decision can be made. We make lists of what we need or want, and then there's less chance of deviating from plans. Making decisions about eating out is difficult and usually results in someone being upset that they didn't get to eat what they wanted, or we'll switch quite rapidly between alters who want different things until someone manages to stay in control. This sort of thing has definitely gotten us some strange looks when suddenly what we wanted originally isn't what we end up asking for, or our accent or tone may change through the sentences. Thankfully, the main disagreements, like what we wear when going out, is something that happens away from the public.

*

AMELIA JOUBERT
Amelia was diagnosed with 12
personalities in 2013 at age 15

My alters do have disagreements in public, but they are usually small, things like what to eat in a restaurant or what shirt to buy at a store. I once saw a post by someone with DID that said "I don't understand the stereotype that people with DID could be killers. Just deciding what to eat for dinner starts an internal civil war. You really think we could plan a murder?" That quote is so true; everything with DID is a negotiation. Although we debate a lot, other people can't really tell. To people who don't know we have DID, we probably just seem very indecisive. It's not like we talk out loud to one another, or switch to talk, like it's portrayed in some movies. I hear my alters in my head, and I can communicate with them internally. Sometimes if I am alone or slip up, I will talk to them out loud, but it's not like it's portrayed in movies.

*

AMANDA LINEBACK
Amanda was diagnosed with hundreds
of personalities in 2013 at age 31

I have never really feared my alters disagreeing in public. Honestly, I spent most of my life with them disagreeing inside my head. My alters don't keep me housebound, but the fear of people outside my system often keeps me from going out. Social situations and crowds make me so nervous that it is often impossible to participate in activities.

I used to worry that my littles would come out and try to play with my kids at a school function or in a toy store. My psychologist taught me about making a contract that is agreed to and signed by everyone. Our first agreement and number one rule that trumps all situations is: all outside and inside children are to be kept safe at all times. This means the children are to be kept safe from physical, spiritual, emotional, sexual, or verbal abuse. We also agreed that no one would be exposed to anything that is outside their age range, for any reason. Lola, who is three, loves to talk to everyone. If there are toys, candy, pets, children, or anything sparkly in a store, she will come out to play. She loves to ask questions and see how everything works. She even tries to give her opinion during adult conversations. Thankfully, I can feel her out front before she says anything, and I can stop her from trying to adult.

There have been times when I went shopping with friends and spent three hours in the same store. I would keep going around the store looking at all the same stuff because someone new would come to the front, which means they're seeing everything for the first time. My friends are patient and they know about my DID, so as long as nobody is on a time schedule, they just shop right along with whoever is out at the moment.

*

JANE MACDONALD
Jane was diagnosed with 3 personalities in
2014 at age 35, and currently has 6 alters

My alters are generally never out at the same time, so I don't have to worry about arguments in public. Many are not even aware of one another. However, the fear of having even just one alter come out in public, of losing time, of not being aware of or able to control what they might do or say, is often enough to keep me housebound most of the time.

*

CRYSTALIE MATULEWICZ
Crystalie was diagnosed with dissociative
identity disorder in 2015 at age 29

Public disagreements have never been an issue. I'm not saying that it hasn't happened. I've never been aware of it, and no one on the outside has ever told me about it. My parts do disagree, but they have them on the inside. It's safer that way. I try to keep my communication with my parts on the inside as well, so I don't find myself in public talking out loud to people who no one else can see.

There is a lot of confusion when I am out shopping. I often find myself standing in the same section for a long time. I'll pick up something, put it down, and then pick up something different. I worry about the looks I get from people. It's very difficult to make a decision when other parts have influence as well.

My parts have different likes and dislikes so it's difficult at times to agree on something, and it usually ends up with me leaving emptyhanded. I don't really fear a public disagreement. I just don't see it happening. If it does, I guess we'll just manage it the way we manage everything else, and go with the flow. I would never let the fear keep me, and us, from living.

*

ALICIA PETTIS
Alicia was diagnosed with 40
personalities in 2015 at age 16

My alters have had disagreements in public before, and I did get dirty looks, but I've learned to live with it over time. I can't control my alters enough to have them not argue. People argue all the time, so why can't my alters argue, even if they argue with each other? I used to stay locked in my room for fear that someone would judge me, but then I realized that my alters are going to leave my room and argue wherever they are, so why should I close up my life when it's a part of who I am? They won't argue around children because of the arguing I had when I was younger. That's one of their rules: if children are around, they keep it to themselves until afterward. They don't want kids to see the arguments.

*

SUNSHINE PURCELL
Denise was diagnosed with 17
personalities in 1995 at age 30

Yes, there have been disagreements in public. To the outside world it looks like I'm talking to myself and, of course, crazy. Or the little ones become excited if they see a toy or a snack they might want. I rarely go alone, because there's nothing worse than getting to a checkout only to find odd things in the cart and not enough money to pay for them. So most of my time is housebound.

I do go to therapy once a week for an hour, and once a month I see the psychiatrist for an update. Having DID limits a lot of activity and interaction, but it's nothing to be scared about. If more people would try to understand why we are like this, it's really quite unique. If I didn't have it, I would love to study it from the outside in, but I would listen to what is being said. Most of us who have this are very smart, talented and just want a normal life. Our alters want a normal life but understand that we have only one body. It's hard to think that my real age is fifty, but I have a little girl in me who *is* me, but has a different name and is five years old. I have a lot of inner children, and all this could have been avoided by love and protecting us as children.

*

ERICKA REEVE
Ericka was diagnosed with over 25
personalities in 2013 at age 26

I was never aware of them until more recently, and while I do stress (unrealistically) about it at times, I know logically that just won't happen more than very rarely, if ever. It's not what they do. Not aloud, anyway. I've spent twenty-eight years with the "something will always happen mentality." Because, honestly, it always does! Always. I prefer my house, but that's where some of them come out. But, you guessed it, they leave the house. And I socialize. They help me to maintain the appearance of normality. We hate the word, but I just don't have a better one. Typical doesn't really cover it, so "normal" is what I say.

*

CHRIS ROBIN
Chris was diagnosed with at least
7 personalities in 2013 at age 49

I learned at a very young age that either in public or private, I was going to have to learn how to have the conversations go on in my

159

head. I used to think that everyone had these voices in their heads, sort of like intuition. I'm learning that I have DID and these parts have shown up in all areas of my life, both private and public. I was able to compartmentalize and be the person I needed to be for the situation, and I had a person in my life who understood that I was different in different situations, and acted differently in public and private. Now that Beth is gone, it is more difficult to control those parts of me who disagree or argue with everything I do.

I used to have a way to communicate all the various feelings and actions of my parts with my partner. In turn, she would help me interpret the world and decipher the actions and reactions of others around me, as well as the various parts of me. Now that she is gone, I am learning that I have to find my own ways to allow all the parts of me to interact with the world. The only way I can cope with arguments or disagreements is to remove myself from the situation, or simply go numb and have no reaction whatsoever. These are probably not very healthy ways of dealing with conflict, but that is what has helped.

It is lonely and isolating because there is no longer anyone who truly understands what is going on in all aspects of my life. I am learning better coping skills and what to do when I am triggered. I am learning to reach out for help and finding a core support group who is compassionate and not too judgmental. When I stay within my routines and schedules, I can usually keep all the parts of me satisfied. But when I get out of those routines and do very unpredictable things socially, I have virtually no idea if a part of me will take over, and that has become scarier and more debilitating.

*

QUINN ROSE
Quinn was diagnosed with 9
personalities in 2016 at age 21

Uh, I don't know. I have never experienced this myself, since I black out when my parts are out.

*

AYA SAKURA
Aya has been living with 7
personalities since childhood

I'm a bit scared of having an argument with my alters in public, because I have a tendency to talk out loud to them while arguing or even just talking. Since I really want to fit in with everyone, I am very scared that people will think I've gone mental, or that I'll have to explain why I'm talking. I mostly try to avoid an argument. Luckily, the only time an argument or disagreement in public could occur is when we are able to talk to each other, which only happens if we are co-conscious.

If you compare my body to a car, then the one who is out is the driver, and the alter who is in the passenger seat is co-conscious with the driver. While in the passenger seat, you can take the wheel to some degree if you want to, and you are also able to talk to the driver and see, hear and experience everything that happens to the driver. The farther back in the car you are, the less co-conscious you are with the driver (and the passenger), and the less you hear and see and are heard if you talk to the driver or the passenger. In the trunk of the car, you don't see, hear or experience anything, and you aren't co-conscious with anyone at all.

Brianna isn't co-conscious with me very often. When she is out, she tends to completely shut me down so that I am in the trunk and can't get co-conscious with her. We don't have very much contact other than through mailing and notes. She's very different from me and has other preferences and needs than I do. Most of the time she is complaining about my choices or about the stuff I do. This results in quite a few arguments when we are being co-conscious. If this happens in public, I always try to stop whatever she's complaining about. This way I can avoid an argument. If I can't stop, for whatever reason, I ignore her as best I can, and talk about it later. The only downside to this is that she gets very angry if she's being ignored, as she is used to always getting her way. I think this is also the reason we don't really have a good relationship.

Clive is regularly co-conscious with me, and we don't get in arguments very much. If I'm out and he is co-conscious, he just tells me what he thinks and lets me decide what I am going to do. When he thinks the situation is getting dangerous or risky, he takes over and comes out and pushes me to the background, and eventually shut me down if needed to protect me. I mostly get pushed to the back seat, so I can get a little information like a sight, sound, the details, or the outline of what happened. Clive doesn't allow others to be co-conscious with him very much. When he does, it's mostly Brianna whom he allows. He's dominant and stable when he's out.

*

MATTHEW SANCHEZ
Matthew was diagnosed with 8
personalities in 2015 at age 16

We rarely disagree on things unless they're very important or sudden. Occasionally we will fight over which candy to get at the movies, but that just results in getting more candy. If something deeply bothers us and we disagree, it can send us into a bad place. We argue in the headspace while our body goes on autopilot and just stands there staring into space. Our communication is improving every day. Thankfully, we can do everything a singlet can do outside of our home.

*

FLOSS SCOTT
Floss was diagnosed with at least
4 personalities in 2016 at age 48

I've had to control my aggressive alter from coming out, because she is uncontrollable. I keep her under control by making sure I don't put myself in the situation for her to come out. If she's close to the front, my sisters know how to calm her down. But she's been locked away for well over twenty years.

*

PAULA SUNDWALL
Paula was diagnosed with dissociative amnesia in 2006 at age
36 and diagnosed with at least 4 personalities in 2014 at age 44

There are very few things I fear happening in public. I've never even considered my alters disagreeing because of the wall between us. I'm not privy to the goings-on with them, so I'm not burdened with that particular worry. My alters have done lots of things in public that other people might find embarrassing or shameful, but it is what it is and there's nothing I can do about it. If someone at the grocery store were to ask me why I was crying while shopping the day before, and refused to talk to anyone, I can say either that I wasn't feeling well, or I can tell him or her the truth, depending on the mood I'm in and how much time I have.

*

KERRYJANE VOTH
Kerryjane was diagnosed with
35 alters in 2013 at age 53

Ha ha ha!!! Yes, yes, yes!!! The fear of losing control of what appears to others as my emotions can be debilitating. It has caused me to develop agoraphobia as well. I once went to a social barbecue. While getting ready, I was sensing some pretty strong resistance by some of my alters, while sensing that others really wanted to attend. We were not in group agreement when we left the house. Not long after arriving, when I realized nobody was talking to me, the body started to experience anxiety and panic. Some of my alters felt like we were being ignored, so I decided to reach out and ask a question and start a friendly conversation. The person I approached wasn't paying attention and didn't respond to my question. One alter jumped on it right away, saying, "See?! This is why we don't like coming to things like this!" Another alter tried to calm him down, and a third alter start crying.

The person I approached spun around full of apologies and joined the conversation, thinking I was speaking to her. But she wasn't part of the conversation at all. The alters were not talking to her, only to each other. By the time tears started rolling down my cheeks, I was on my way to the elevator. I needed a quick retreat to calm everyone down and to regroup.

Needless to say, the next time I saw the poster for another barbecue, my alters screamed, "No f*** way! We're not going to that again!" Days later I had to try to smooth it over with the person I had approached at the barbecue, since she didn't understand what had happened and felt really bad that she had upset me.

*

Can You See Us?
BY SCARLET JOUBERT

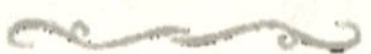

You see her but do you see me?

You don't see the cheerful girl with the purple hair.

You don't see the man who comforts and takes care of us.

You don't see the sassy southern redhead or her sassy little girl.

The quiet boy who watches over us

and has an amazing talent for art.

The little 6-year-old girl who just wants candy and to play.

You can't see the little boy who only wants to make everyone

happy or the scared little girl he tries so hard to make happy.

The young teenage girl who watches after these kids.

The skater boy and the punk rock girl

who never want to be apart.

You don't see us but we're here.

You don't know our names but we exist.

One day maybe you'll know and

you'll see us and believe in us.

Maybe one day.

*

CHAPTER EIGHT

The System within

> During the day, I was a puzzle with innumerable pieces. One piece made my family a nourishing breakfast. Another piece ferried the kids to school and to soccer practice. A third piece managed to trip to the grocery store. There was also a piece that wanted to sleep for eighteen hours a day and the piece that woke up shaking from yet another nightmare. -SUZIE BURKE

Some individuals living with dissociative identity disorder have a system or inner world where the alters reside when not in control of the body. Others don't have a system or inner world that they are aware of. How would you describe your inner world or system?

*

ADRIANNE ALLEN-LANG
Adrianne was diagnosed with 10
personalities in 2015 at age 18

Our inner world begins as a long hallway. In the beginning it was a dark and ominous hallway, but now as more alters come out of hiding it gets brighter and brighter. It resembles a hotel hallway; long, with a door at the very end, and about ten doors on either side of it. There are doors all along that lead to the rooms of my others, which I can't access. A few doorways lead to the common room, which is constantly changing and is a lot like the Room of Requirement in Harry Potter. Another door leads to the tower out back where our most violent alter lives. The door at the end leads to the library where all our memories and experiences are stored. Myrnin, our vampire, is the keeper of these books of memories, and lives in the library permanently.

I am aware of what is going on with seven of the ten alters. The other three rarely front, so I haven't gotten to bond with them enough to be co-conscious. Any alter can kick me back to the inner world when they're fronting though, if they wish to. Th e feeling is similar to having not slept for days on end. Everything is blurry, disproportionate, and time feels unreal and fake, like a dream. It's like you're watching what's going on but with no control, like being on autopilot. We don't decide who comes out; others just do things when they're needed. For example, during my art class a few days ago, I had a bad artist block and couldn't think of anything, so Anna came out. Within an hour, she had an entire watercolor and ink piece seventy-five percent completed.

I was getting angry in traffic this morning due to a pileup, and Keegan came out so I didn't end up screaming at someone. They don't just come out for trauma-related needs; they help me in my day-to-day life.

*

GAIL BUSWELL
Gail was diagnosed with 13
personalities in 2002 at age 24

My inner world used to be beautiful. It was filled with happy places and all the things that made us happy. Now it is a very dark and scary place. It is so busy all the time, with very little peace. Everybody is fighting to be heard, and my littles spend a lot of time in a state of distress. I have no control of who fronts and for how long. I am co-conscious with very few of my others at the moment.

*

KATT HART
Katt was diagnosed with hundreds
of personalities in 2011 at age 20

The inner world where the alters live is large and complicated. There's a huge ocean with various islands and some buildings on the islands. Most of us don't know much about other islands, since we can communicate only with the ones on the island we live on. But we hear about the others a little bit from our partner, and some alters have drawn maps or written details about it.

On the central island, the one that's active more than the others, there are five buildings that people live in, a beach and a play area. There's also a forest and a beach, and there's a dark scary cave, but we don't venture into that since it's dark and seems dangerous.

When one of us is out, we can tell what some are doing if they're around us inside, but we can only guess about the ones who aren't near us. We have fairly good communication with a lot of people on our island and can usually tell what someone is doing, or we might know someone inside who can see what's happening. It's a large group of alters though, so it's unusual for many to know what's happening unless we tell them about it later, or show them the memories.

We rarely decide who's out. If we really need or want someone to be out, then our partner will try to help us by calling the alter out, usually calling his or her name over and over, talking about things specifically about them, or watching or listening to something they enjoy. There's no real time limit on how long someone can be out for, though. It depends on when someone else wants to come out, or if we have an appointment that someone else would be better suited for. We're not very organized and don't work on a schedule. It works all right for us, since we don't have a job or children.

*

AMELIA JOUBERT
Amelia was diagnosed with 12
personalities in 2013 at age 15

I'm not sure how big our inner world is, but I've seen parts of the mansion and the town. The mansion is on top of a hill and the main twelve of us live in it. It has bedrooms for us, a living room, kitchen, playroom, and other rooms you would find in any house. We also have a room called the viewing room that allows us to communicate with whoever is out. At the bottom of the hill is a town that has an apartment building where the insiders live. The town also has several stores, including a tattoo parlor and a hair salon. Most people in the town have a job, but money is not used in our inner world.

*

AMANDA LINEBACK
Amanda was diagnosed with hundreds
of personalities in 2013 at age 31

My inner world is in the middle of a magical forest where faeries, unicorns, and mystical creatures live. Our house is hidden inside a big tree that has been enchanted so only people with pure intentions can enter. When you first enter there's a big hallway lined with huge mahogany doors. The doors have locks with no keys, and can only be opened by answering a secret question. At the very end of the hall, a big black door is guarded by four giants. I have only been in the very first door in this hallway, and I have no idea what the others have behind them. When you enter the door that leads to my community, you immediately smell freshly baked cookies. Open doorways line the beautifully carpeted hallways, and everything feels warm and inviting. One room has quiet classical music playing; inside, mothers are holding and singing to their babies. Grandmothers are also holding babies and rocking them to sleep.

The next room is full of tables, art supplies, and coloring books. The children's artwork is displayed on the walls. Some rooms serve as recreational rooms, and are broken down by age groups. These rooms are supervised by adults who volunteer to take care of the little ones when their parents aren't home. Farther down there's a door that leads to an outside patio. There is a huge garden with vegetables and fruit, and an enormous concrete slab dedicated to sidewalk chalk. In a separate hallway there are doors that lead to the home of each family. There is a gymnasium that holds meetings and recreational events.

There are many hidden passages and rooms that can be entered only by certain people. We have to be careful about who hears what we say, and make sure we aren't being spied on by the watchers. If you get caught committing treason, they throw you in the dungeon.

*

JANE MACDONALD
Jane was diagnosed with 3 personalities in
2014 at age 35, and currently has 6 alters

Unlike many people with DID, I do not have an inner world. I don't really have any idea what the other alters do when they are not out. To me, they just kind of disappear. Very occasionally I can sense or be aware of what the out alters are doing. A person in an online DID group once described it as being similar to being in a vehicle. Sometimes I am the driver, and have complete awareness and control while my alters are the passengers. Other times I am in the passenger seat. I can see what is happening and can try to influence what the alter who is driving is doing. I can even try to grab the wheel when necessary. However, ultimately what happens is up to that alter. Other times I am in the back seat and have little awareness of what is going on with little or no influence. Most of the time I am in the trunk. I cannot hear, see, or have any understanding of what is going on. I am completely in the dark. I cannot talk to or reason with the alter who is out. I cannot influence what is happening. This is what it is like for me the vast majority of the time. Unfortunately, I seem to have very little to no control over who takes over and decides to drive. I do not decide who is out, or for how long. All I can do is go along for the ride—and hope that nothing horrible happens.

*

CRYSTALIE MATULEWICZ
Crystalie was diagnosed with dissociative
identity disorder in 2015 at age 29

I didn't have much of an inner world for a long time, it just consisted of darkness. When I joined DID support groups online, I read about how others experience an inner world, and how they had all these beautiful houses with rooms, gardens, toys, and lovely things. I had none of that. I had a giant black hole of nothingness.

I spent so much time trying to create a safe space for my parts on the outside. I bought books for all different reading levels, stuffed animals, coloring books, and toys. I bought a punching bag and set it up for my teenaged parts to release their anger. I put all my energy into making sure my parts had something meaningful for them in the outside world. I never thought of creating anything on the inside. My therapist said an inner world could help give my parts a place to go, so they could feel safe.

I'm admittedly not very good at visualization, so the thought of conceptualizing this whole inner world in my head was daunting, and at times overwhelming. It is something I am working on. I don't have access to the inner world myself. When I dissociate, I just fade into the background, so to speak. I'm not able to go all the way inside to their world. I try to ask my parts what they need on the inside, and help them make it. Eventually I hope to get to a place where my parts don't have to stay in darkness any more.

As far as the parts inside of my inner world, my alters, we all have varying levels of co-consciousness. There are a few of my parts who I am co-conscious with. When they are present, I am also there, sometimes in control and sometimes not. Think of it like being in a car. We are both sitting in the front, and both can see everything that is going on. But one of us is at the wheel driving the car and the other is a passenger. Sometimes I am the one driving. Other times I'm riding shotgun. Even though I can see what's going on and what I'm doing, I don't have control over what's going on; another part does.

There are times when a part is out, and I have no awareness of anything going on, outside or inside. I feel like I'm just in a haze. This tends to happen when I am under extreme stress. I don't know what goes on when I am completely dissociated. Sometimes someone on the outside asks me about something I did during that time, and I struggle to find an answer.

I'm still working on connecting with the parts of my system, so I don't really know. A time may come when I gain more awareness and co-consciousness, or not. I do let my parts know that they can come out in therapy if they need to talk. I try to encourage my parts to stay inside when I am doing grownup things like work and school, since many are little. I read books to my younger parts to let them know they are safe and help them understand what's going on. I want my parts to know that they are valid, but I also know that we live in a world that doesn't readily understand what being multiple means. Most times it is safer to be on the inside.

*
ALICIA PETTIS
Alicia was diagnosed with 40
personalities in 2015 at age 16

My inner world is both small and large. In the middle of it is a white building that resembles either a very large apartment, hotel, or a semi-large hospital. Each alter has their own room that they decorate to their liking. There's also a large family room where all my alters, me included, can hang out if we prefer not to stay in our room. A room for our littles is just off the family room; they feel safe and secure there when the system is in chaos. Not far from the family room is a giant room with wooden floors where dances are held once a month to relieve any stress that we might be going through. Outside is a giant oak tree that holds a treehouse, which belongs to Sammie. You're allowed in only if he says so. Next to that is a playground with sand for the littles to play in. Surrounding that are woods. Most alters walk through the woods on the trail for fear of getting lost, but if one was to go off the trail, he or she would find the chambers, where the harmful and dark three are locked away.

When one alter is out, I'm either in the dark room where I can't see or hear anything, or in the system's inner world. The only way for me to know what an alter is doing while they're out is for me to be co-conscious or paying really close attention in the inner world. Since I normally get sent to the dark room, I don't know what they're doing while they're out. An alter will stay out for as long as he or she feels like they should. If they feel it's been too long but I'm not mentally stable enough to handle being out, another alter takes over. We have rules and everyone obeys them; that's how our system works.

*

SUNSHINE PURCELL
Denise was diagnosed with 17
personalities in 1995 at age 30

My inner world is a world of its own. I'm not aware of what is going on with who, what, and why unless there is either evidence, like a tea party doll set, crayons and a coloring picture, or a burn mark from the glue gun. The biggest clue is the stuffed animals the little ones carry with them when feeling alone or scared.

I seem to just check out. I don't remember anything and I don't know where I've been. There isn't an island in my world to go to. They are pretty good at knowing if something is very important and needs to be done. They have inner communication with each other, and make plans accordingly. If the artist has to be out, then maybe later the little ones can watch a movie or play. It took a lot of trust from certain people to allow them to be who they are. There came a lot of trial and error, and still I wish I knew what was going on. I feel cheated a lot, but getting mad isn't going to help me. I just do the best I can, sometimes to a fault, and take it day by day.

*

ERICKA REEVE
Ericka was diagnosed with over 25
personalities in 2013 at age 26

I don't get to decide who is out and when, nor do I determine the duration. Things were bad (putting it *very* mildly) for a long time. I'm only recently aware of my diagnosis and am trying to work through it. It *is* work. Struggling can be defined in various ways and degrees, but

I say *struggling.* To state it simply, they just come in and help, which is kind of the point of what DID is in its most basic definition. I cannot describe my inner world. It doesn't seem to exist specifically in that way, not for me, not yet. I'm sure it's there in some way for them, but for me it's just not.

*

CHRIS ROBIN
Chris was diagnosed with at least
7 personalities in 2013 at age 49

For most of my life, I didn't know that parts of me were working and doing things for me. It hasn't been until now that therapy and education about DID is helping me to recognize how the different parts of me have been taking over and affecting various aspects of my life. I just knew that I acted and responded and felt differently in different situations.

As a teacher, the daily work structure and routine allowed those parts who were needed to do that work, and to participate in that part of my life. But hanging out with friends or family brought out other parts to help me deal with the unpredictability of those relationships. It became comfortable to simply make sure that those groups of people didn't interact, and no one would know that I was acting and behaving differently in different situations.

The only constant in all parts of my world was my partner, Beth. She accepted me as I am and loved me anyway. Her death has had a major impact on my life. My biggest fear has always been that others would see these changes though I've learned to hide them pretty well.

For half of my life, my various parts had been able to come and go as needed, and really only in times of severe stress or trauma has it been more difficult to control or understand why one part deserted me or showed up unexpectedly. I know that at times when I don't get enough sleep or enough rest, and when those parts don't have ways to release their energy or when I don't take my medication, my inner world becomes chaotic and overwhelming. I am still learning to recognize when one alter or another is present, and am beginning to open more communication with them so we can learn to work together rather than separately. This is a new concept for me. I am just now really beginning to understand that I have an inner world. It has taken the form of a house with various rooms, floors, and a conference room that helps open the lines of communication. I am learning that each of the parts are in me, and what they have been holding on to for me, or protecting me from.

*

QUINN ROSE
Quinn was diagnosed with 9
personalities in 2016 at age 21

I don't have an inner world. It's just dark, and then a lot of time has passed, sometimes days. I always keep a calendar.

*

AYA SAKURA
Aya has been living with 7
personalities since childhood

For me, the inner world means floating in a black space. There is no gravity. I normally get no sensory input. Sometimes I get flashes of what's going on outside, sometimes I remember certain memories of myself or of my alters, but mostly I get nothing.

When my alters aren't out, they are in a city. We call it London because my alters consider themselves British, but the city is just a representation of a very big city. It has resemblances to London as well as Amsterdam, Paris, New York, and my hometown. Basically, it's the world in a city, if that makes sense. They've got their own life and history there, which also shaped their personalities. My alters are able to do whatever they want in the inner world.

In the inner world, Clive and Brianna are married and have a band together with a few friends. Brianna is the vocalist, while Clive plays the synthesizer and keyboard. They write lyrics together and after the other band members have given their approval, they sit as a group to write the music. They live together in an apartment and have a studio where they record and practice with their band.

Brianna is from a wealthy family and has very good looks. She is doing modeling work. Her family passed away, so she moved in with Clive. Because she's so wealthy, she is used to having maids around doing all the work. Clive is also a writer. He writes columns, reviews, articles, literally everything. He also does all the housework. He has a sister, Sabrina (yes, she used to be an alter), but she moved out of London.

In the inner world, Alice is a very good friend of Brianna and Clive. She moved out of London to study computer sciences. Brianna recently got a message from Alice saying she had graduated and was planning on moving back. Makah and Lucy are very good friends in the inner world. Makah also is friends with Sabrina, while Lucy is friends with Alice. I don't know if they still are in London. I sometimes am able to see a bit of the inner world, but that's only when I'm very dissociated and have no clue who I am. I don't really know how our inner world works.

*

FLOSS SCOTT
Floss was diagnosed with at least
4 personalities in 2016 at age 48

My inner world feels like my life has been torn apart. There's been so much trauma. I'm constantly feeling that I have to be strong, but really I'm weak and shattered. My heart has been broken one too many times, but I'm not giving up on myself.

*

PAULA SUNDWALL
Paula was diagnosed with dissociative amnesia in 2006 at age
36 and diagnosed with at least 4 personalities in 2014 at age 44

Secretive. Hidden. Clandestine. My alters do not speak to me. I do not hear voices. We are walled off from each other out of fear. When I first began experiencing severe disassociation at around age fourteen, I would have panic attacks as a way of stopping my body from being taken over, which was my greatest fear. This lasted for over twenty years and, I suspect, trained my alters to come out only when I'm asleep, extremely fatigued, or very distracted. Now that I have overcome my fear and my panic attacks are under control, I would very much like to know what is going on in there. I am currently seeking help from someone who may be able to teach me to open the lines of communication.

*

KERRYJANE VOTH
Kerryjane was diagnosed with
35 alters in 2013 at age 53

My inner world has vast open spaces, rooms with closed doors, terra firma locations, and a spaceship with a control room like the USS Enterprise. My inner world is filled with patterns and colors, tastes and smells, lights, and lots of dark. Up and down and a nothingness space, all-consuming of time to infinity. It is a universe that's as vast within as it is without, where I can travel anywhere in time or space.

*

Nothing
BY SUNSHINE

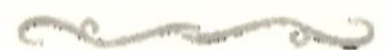

To awake Christmas morning
awaiting presents under the tree
Would be so very wonderful,
maybe ones for me?

Maybe a new baby doll
with eyes that open wide,
And when you hug her close to you
"I love you" sounds bellow from inside,

Or maybe a stuffed gingerbread
that's so soft to the touch
And each night before I go to bed
I'll say "Ginger, I love you so much."

Or maybe a new dress with
velvet ribbons trimmed with lace
And as I look into the mirror
A smile appears on my face,

You're beautiful my darling,
my sweet baby girl
As my daddy picks me up
and gives me a little twirl,

With stockings filled with candy
and everything so brand new
Only in my wildest dreams
that finally have come true,

But as the light shines through
and morning says it's here
I awake again to find nothing,
and again nothing was my greatest fear.

CHAPTER NINE

Making Arrangements

A person continually deals with not remembering
what one has said or done. Thus, the person with
DID must be quick with inferences and cover-ups.
— ELIZABETH HOWELL

Living with others who share the same body usually requires some sort of agreement or arrangement. This helps to plan and manage activities of daily life with some sort of predictability and dependability for everyone involved. What arrangements do you have in place among alters to help your daily routine go smoothly?

*

ADRIANNE ALLEN-LANG
Adrianne was diagnosed with 10
personalities in 2015 at age 18

We don't have any arrangements in place. It's taken a long time for us to get to where we are, cooperation wise, and everyone has mutual understanding and respect with one another for the body's daily routine and needs. Occasionally we'll have an issue or two when someone is having a bad day and hijacks the body from the routine. If it's something minor, that night we'll sit down within the inner world while the body sleeps and discuss it. But if it's a severe hijacking—like a few months ago when Keegan went to go driving across the country unlicensed—then Nurse and Allie have a kill switch which immediately pushes back whoever is fronting, and pushes out someone else, usually Anna or Kitty. Everyone gets along most of the time. As with any family, there are fights and disagreements, but there are also so many good times and gorgeous memories.

*

KATT HART
Katt was diagnosed with hundreds
of personalities in 2011 at age 20

We don't have much of a routine, but if cleaning or cooking needs to be done and alters who can't or won't do that are out, then we'll try to coax them out or ask our partner to help call to them to see if they'll come. We have very few rules, and so far none of them have been broken that I can remember. But if anyone were to break a rule, there absolutely would be consequences, but it depends on what they did.

While we don't all get along, most will at least work together. Since most understand that we share this body and this life, we may as well make it as comfortable as possible, and fighting would only complicate things. So we're very lucky to have most people working as a team wherever possible. Our partner has been a gigantic help in this area by reminding everyone of this when anyone starts to rebel.

*

AMELIA JOUBERT
Amelia was diagnosed with 12
personalities in 2013 at age 15

We have several system rules. One is that we can't monopolize the time. Anyone who wants time, we have to give it to him or her. I always joke that people with DID should get more time in the day. The littles want time to play, we need time to do schoolwork, and everyone wants time to do things they enjoy. Nine different people, not including the kids, want time to watch their show, read their book, and do hobbies they enjoy. Having DID means negotiation is key. For the kids, we have rules like any other kid would have, like a bedtime, and they can have sweets only when adults say it's okay.

*

AMANDA LINEBACK
Amanda was diagnosed with hundreds
of personalities in 2013 at age 31

We make sure that the outside children are taken care of, and other than that we do not have a routine.

*

JANE MACDONALD
Jane was diagnosed with 3 personalities in
2014 at age 35, and currently has 6 alters

We don't have any arrangements in place, largely because of a lack of awareness among alters. There is not much communication between my personalities and myself. Although I have attempted to initiate communication by talking to them (whether they listen is another matter) or leaving notes, these efforts have been largely unacknowledged and unreciprocated.

Most days I am in control and things go relatively smoothly. Other days I can be completely unaware of what happened that day, how things went, or what was said or done. I have to rely on information that others in my life tell me: friends, my employer, coworkers, etc. If an alter wants or needs to come out, I am not yet able to control that or prevent it from happening. I just have to hope that my daily routine and other activities are not interrupted much. I hope one day to develop enough of a system of communication and cooperation to ensure that things like routines and daily functioning go smoothly, but I am not there yet.

In terms of consequences, I don't have any in place, largely because of lack of awareness of what my alters do when they are out. It's also hard to have consequences for the older and more aggressive alters, particularly Kali, who is the self-destructive one. Honestly, I don't know what kind of consequences to make for an alter who cuts me or otherwise harms the body, particularly since I am not aware of what age she is. The youngest alters don't usually misbehave (to my understanding, at least), so there isn't much need for consequences. I do offer the littlest one, Clara, candy or toys sometimes like when she doesn't come out during therapy, but then I have to rely on my psychiatrist to tell me if she was out during our session or not.

Not all of my alters are aware of each other, and those who are do not always get along. Kali, in particular, is angry and hates everyone else, including me (Jane). She does things to hurt the body, and others who are aware of her, particularly Clara, are scared of her. Angela can also be difficult to get along with and often acts out by saying things she shouldn't, but for the most part sticks to herself.

I've heard people describe their system as being like a family, and so naturally there are disagreements. Mine is more like a group of total strangers of different ages and interests residing in the same body and mind. Just as I don't get along with every person I meet, my alters don't always get along either. It's tough sharing the same space with people you don't know and don't have anything in common with. At times it feels like living in a college dorm: some people stick to themselves and rarely come out of their rooms, while others are out and about, and get along with each other. And still others are around yet dislike one another. It's not perfect, but then life never is. I just learn to deal with things as they come up.

*

CRYSTALIE MATULEWICZ
Crystalie was diagnosed with dissociative
identity disorder in 2015 at age 29

Daily routine is something we are still working on. Before, I didn't take control over anything. There were no arrangements. I gave up control to whoever took it, because I was just so exhausted most of the time. It was chaos. I have some medical issues that require me to take medications multiple times a day. I couldn't remember whether I took the medication. Sometimes I didn't take it at all, and sometimes I ended up taking it twice. I couldn't always remember if we ate that day. It was a disaster.

After working on some of the aspects of my DID in therapy, I realized that I needed to take control and put some kind of system in place for us. My therapist encouraged me to keep a daily log. Every hour or so I would check in and make a note of what I was doing, how I was feeling, and if anything significant was happening. I did this every day for a couple of months. Doing that helped me realize what was going on in my day-to-day life, as I was in and out of dissociation and couldn't remember a lot of things. Now I have a better awareness of the times when I am most dissociated, and what emotions and experiences tie into that.

I keep a planner. Every Saturday I write everything that needs to be done in the coming week with specific dates, times, and locations: work shifts, therapy sessions, doctor appointments, medication regimens, meetings, homework assignments, even when to do laundry. This way everyone knows what has to be done. There have been instances when a part got us to work or took us to therapy because I wasn't fully present. The schedule allows us to keep a routine, no matter what part is out.

There have been times when I had to schedule even the most basic tasks, like eating a meal. Some of my parts, as well as I, have disordered eating patterns related to childhood trauma. This results in a lot of disagreement over meals, and sometimes not wanting to eat at all. During the last few years I have lost a substantial amount of weight and had issues with malnutrition, so starvation only makes that worse. I need to take vitamins every day which helps, but food is still a necessity. To keep us somewhat healthy, I try to prep meals ahead of time, and set reminders in our schedule to eat dinner. While one meal a day isn't ideal, it's what I can handle right now. I have an app on my phone that reminds us to log in our meal every day. It helps to keep track when it's hard to remember. There are still struggles here and there, but everyone knows that eating every day is important, and keeps us from ending up in the hospital again.

Fortunately, most of our system gets along. Of course, it's not all peace, love, and agreement. There are disagreements and differences in opinion, just as there are among people who aren't multiple. The only difference is that our disagreements take place on the inside, and not on the outside.

I try to approach our system as if we were a team, ultimately having to work together so we can be better as a whole. We need each other in order to run smoothly.

*

ALICIA PETTIS
Alicia was diagnosed with 40
personalities in 2015 at age 16

One rule we have in our system is that the littles aren't allowed out while driving, when one of us is taking an important exam or quiz, or during intense films. Also, when it comes to relationships with outside sources, there must be a conversation with my current partner and me. There are many more rules and if an alter breaks one, consequences are dealt. Depending on the severity of the rule that's broken, the consequences aren't too severe. Rule-breaking used to happen all the time, but after my first protector and co-host stepped up to her role, everyone began obeying the rules. Other than that, most of my alters get along very well aside from the harmful three who are locked away. Like most people, they have creative differences and will get into arguments. But besides that, they all get along very well.

*

SUNSHINE PURCELL
Denise was diagnosed with 17
personalities in 1995 at age 30

It kind of just fell into place. I'm usually out first in the morning, but not always. Sometimes the little ones will wander downstairs and tell my fiancé they had a bad dream or that I had a seizure and have a headache. There really can't be consequences in my case, because if one does something they shouldn't have, it affects us all. For example, if Boots wants to go out dancing and drink too much, she doesn't have the ability to understand poor judgment or consequences, because she's fragmented—not a whole personality. But the next day, we all suffer from the hangover and what else might have happened.

I have one who does daily duties. The Mother takes care of dinners and entertainment. The Smart One takes care of homework, doctor appointments, insurance companies, school functions. For the most part, they do get along. They might argue, like a family, but there is really not a dislike among any of them. If something is dangerous or not acceptable, they let someone they trust know about it. There is more self-loathing than violence, because of what has happened. But one time Sarah, the five-year-old, wanted to drive. She let one of the older daughters know, and they told her she was too young, that it was dangerous and she needed to wait to come out. That's all it took.

*
ERICKA REEVE
Ericka was diagnosed with over 25
personalities in 2013 at age 26

Our arrangements aren't set in stone. They barely exist. I do not hold consequences over the heads of my parts. They're very capable, more so than I am, or have ever been. They are why I am still breathing, so consequences? No.

That being said, some of us are now working on trying to get along and work together. They do not all get along. Do you get along easily with people who are completely different from you? How would that go if you were trapped in a room with several people you had nothing in common with for twenty or so years? I imagine you'd do anything you could to get through the only exit, regardless of who you had to step on to get there.

*
CHRIS ROBIN
Chris was diagnosed with at least
7 personalities in 2013 at age 49

I am new at all this DID stuff, so I am learning that all my parts don't necessarily know each other. The older parts of me have a hard time dealing with the younger parts, and those arguments and disagreements have caused problems. I am just now beginning to make arrangements or rules. I have been practicing how to come to a meeting place in the house in my head, and when the parts of me are not needed they each have their own comfortable rooms to get away from my world or the other parts. This house and these rooms have had to undergo some remodeling and transforming, and as I learn more about what each part needs to feel safe and comfortable, it is becoming easier to open lines of communication with each part. It is a slow and very scary process, and once you begin to go down the road of understanding, there is no turning around. I have found that you can't unlearn what you find out from your parts. So as painful as this process can be, my therapist is working on helping me understand that it will lead to a healthier, happier life.

*

QUINN ROSE
Quinn was diagnosed with 9
personalities in 2016 at age 21

I have no arrangement with my parts. I have never met my parts, nor can I talk to them.

*

AYA SAKURA
Aya has been living with 7
personalities since childhood

I actually have quite a few arrangements in place, now that I think about it. I just wrote down a few. We actually have more, but it will be a long list, and I can't seem to think of them at the moment. I have an electronic agenda on Google where me and my alters put all our appointments and deadlines with the times, locations and important notes or descriptions. This calendar synchronizes with my phone, so my alters and me are always able to check the schedule. My phone, which is always in my bag or right next to me, is almost always set on sound. I always set a reminder for events half an hour before, since most of the places we go to are within half an hour of traveling time. This way we are able to get everywhere on time, for the most part.

I also have a notebook, Number Two, where we all write down messages, homework for college, deadlines, test dates, and other important stuff that the others need to know. This notebook is also always in my bag or right by my side.

All our stuff lies in a certain place in our room, so that none of us have to search for stuff when there is a need to leave ASAP. My bag almost always contains all the important stuff we need when we go somewhere. It has my phone, wallet, a notebook for when we need paper or whatever, and the notebook Number Two.

To help ground and to know what time it is, I always wear a watch. My alters know it really helps me with recollecting when things happened and to calm myself down, so they also made it part of their morning routine to put it on. It also really helps my alters to check on the time and get going.

My alters both got themselves email addresses. We try to email each other so we can have longer conversations over big topics, and decide things collectively. It is difficult to keep this up, since my alters don't check their email every time they are out and when they don't have internet access. It also happens that they (me as well) are not in the mood to email back, or email at all. I am also a bit slow with emailing back. Brianna doesn't like emailing, so she always sends back just a few lines, no matter how much I write her. I have the best emailing contact with Clive. I think they email each other as well, but I'm not sure.

In case we have messages we need to pass on for the next day, I have a piece of paper lying under my phone. There we write stuff down for the next day, like unconfirmed appointments or things we have to do.

To help feel like ourselves and ground ourselves, we wear a ring, and everyone puts it on the finger they prefer. This also has another function, namely knowing who was out before you. Then I or my alters (me most of the time) can ask that specific person what was going on, or what we missed.

We don't really have many rules, as we are a small system. The main focus of our arrangements is to minimize amnesia. We get along pretty well. Brianna and I fight sometimes, but then Clive comes out. Brianna can be very rebellious, and sometimes breaks rules. Clive handles that most of the time. He puts her back in her place, and then she's angry for a few days. Clive manages us and plans daily activities, and he gives Brianna a lot of time and space to do whatever she wants. That way he keeps her in check.

*

FLOSS SCOTT
Floss was diagnosed with at least
4 personalities in 2016 at age 48

My alters appear when I'm at risk. They all come out at different times, and only when they have to.

Miss Walkover: She's loving, caring and will do anything for anyone. She finds it difficult to say no, and is very weak. She is the main host alter.

Miss Professional. A perfectionist, she's the second main alter.

Miss Protector: She comes out when I'm vulnerable, hurt, upset, or need protecting. She stays until she feels I can cope again.

Miss Aggressive. She's the fighter, and is uncontrollable, but she hasn't been out for over twenty years.

Little Me: She's five years old, and appears after a seizure when I'm feeling embarrassed.

Teen Me: She's twelve, and will appear after a seizure.

*

PAULA SUNDWALL
Paula was diagnosed with dissociative amnesia in 2006 at age
36 and diagnosed with at least 4 personalities in 2014 at age 44

Because of the utter lack of communication, other than the occasional note or Facebook post, there are no arrangements. I get hijacked routinely by my alters. I only know what gets reported back to me by others who have seen me. When an alter takes over, I usually black out completely. Sometimes people can tell the difference between the alters and me, but other times, there is no way to be aware that I am not really there. There is an alter who cries all the time, but does daily chores and things that I have procrastinated on. There is one who wrecked my car regularly, which is why I no longer have a driver's license. This may be the same alter who cuts me and has written suicide notes. So my daily routine is anything but routine. It is unknown territory from one minute to the next.

*

KERRYJANE VOTH
Kerryjane was diagnosed with
35 alters in 2013 at age 53

I start my day as I'm getting ready for bed. Each night I go through a bedtime routine that signals to the nighttime system that it's time to find the Sleepytime alter, and all other alters need to be quiet to get the rest the body needs. The agreement is that when the head hits the pillow, all conversations must stop. I ask that all alters who don't want to sleep go to a quiet place out of earshot and carry on. If anyone has an issue that is pressing, it will be addressed the next day. I agree to provide the system with anything that is requested at bedtime such as food for an empty tummy, teddy bear for the littles, warm blankets or a cool breeze, melatonin to help calm the nighttime system, and earplugs to shut the outside world door so as not to startle the system awake during the night.

When I start to wake, it's agreed that no one is allowed to jump into the body to try to take over. I give the system a whole hour of quietness before even setting foot on the ground. Then the morning routine starts. Wash, dress, walk my service dog, Dax, breakfast, and then a nap. Again, all these activities must be agreed upon by the whole system, and each alter who performs tasks while occupying the body, or there won't be any cooperation.

*

CHAPTER TEN

Determining a Leader

A leader is one who knows the way, goes the way,
and shows the way. -JOHN C. MAXWELL

Although alters and host learn to coexist, sometimes one or more alters can take charge and act as a leader when things become chaotic. When that happens, do you have one leader who acts to restore peace within the system? How do you avoid trouble?

*

ADRIANNE ALLEN-LANG
Adrianne was diagnosed with 10
personalities in 2015 at age 18

No one is in charge; we work as a democratic system majority of the time, but there are a few issues we've had to discuss. Everyone has agreed that I have end-of-day say in some of those issues, one of which is about my son. The only one we seem to ever have severe issues with is Muscle, but he is also mentally unwell, so we don't blame him as such. He lives locked in his tower, but he enjoys the solidarity so it's a win-win situation. If for any reason anyone gets out of control,

Myrnin deals with them. Being a vampire, he drains them of their life force until they pass out, so as to defuse the situation. Once they come to, we all sit down and work out what went wrong.

*

KATT HART
Katt was diagnosed with hundreds
of personalities in 2011 at age 20

We don't have anyone in charge or any single person who's out the most. The adults get to make the final decisions on the bigger things that impact our lives. There are internal meetings between alters, so they can all bring up the things they want or need and they'll try to make a note of it and make arrangements. So when one teen alter wanted his own sketchbook to draw and write his feelings and memories in, we worked together to find one for him to use.

There are a lot of struggles with certain alters. Some want things that aren't realistic, some try to hurt us, and some try to push people away from us. It's all very tiring. Usually when these alters are more active, some of the protector, older alters will try to get them under control and get them to back off until they're willing to cooperate and be reasonable. This doesn't always work, which means we end up with alters snapping at loved ones and starting small fights, or our money gets recklessly spent, or we isolate ourselves. It's an ongoing battle, but we do try to work together!

*

AMELIA JOUBERT
Amelia was diagnosed with 12
personalities in 2013 at age 15

There is no one person who is in charge. The five oldest of us, me, Ahina, Jax, Scarlet, and John are involved in the decision-making for our system. Sometimes May is also involved. We don't decide as a group on everything, but on bigger things we do. For smaller things, like what to have for lunch, people might provide input, but the person who is out will make the ultimate decision. For bigger things, we discuss them before making a decision. For really big things we have a meeting. When a decision can't be made, we take a vote.

*

AMANDA LINEBACK
Amanda was diagnosed with hundreds
of personalities in 2013 at age 31

The boss is the person who programmed us during our abuse. It is something that we are still too scared to discuss.

*

JANE MACDONALD
Jane was diagnosed with 3 personalities in
2014 at age 35, and currently has 6 alters

It's difficult to say that anyone is in charge per se. My situation is very much like a group of strangers all living in the same place. There's no real leader or boss. If I had to pick one, I guess it would be myself, as I'm the one who is out the most and am responsible for making all the decisions. Many of my alters are small children, so they wouldn't be able, and likely wouldn't wish, to be in charge.

I do struggle with alters, but not in terms of making any kind of decisions. I struggle with one alter in particular who is destructive and self-harms a lot. I believe she has also attempted to take her, my, and the other alters' lives a few times. Sadly, there is no communication, and any efforts I make to address her are not reciprocated.

I also often struggle to comfort my littlest alter who seems to always be afraid. I have a bag of items that I keep for her which has things like coloring pages and pencil crayons, teddy bears, a blanket, candy, etc. I am not usually co-conscious with her for long, so it's hard to comfort her directly. The best I can do is have things available and hope that she knows enough to use them when she is out.

*

CRYSTALIE MATULEWICZ
Crystalie was diagnosed with dissociative
identity disorder in 2015 at age 29

For a long time I felt like I wasn't in charge. I am working on that now. It doesn't mean that I am in any way the boss. I would like to work together with my parts. I try to include them in decision-making. I let them know they are being heard, that they are important and valid, and that we are a team. It's much better for all of us if we work together, rather than being in a power struggle and working against each other.

I have a teenage part, Charlie, who believed he was the boss. In many ways he was. He was taking control of the inside all those years when I had no idea what was going on. Our original system leader disappeared after a traumatic incident, and Charlie took over. He led with a lot of anger and hostility. I realized that it was because he was dealing with the effects of his own trauma in the only ways he knew how.

Once I started to work on my DID, I started taking some of the leadership role. I told my parts that I could protect them, and that I could keep them safe and that we weren't in danger. I told Charlie that he didn't have to be in charge anymore, and he can just be a teenager. It's still a struggle sometimes, and he still has a bit of that need to lead in him, but we are finding ways to work together.

*

ALICIA PETTIS
Alicia was diagnosed with 40
personalities in 2015 at age 16

I am not in charge of the system. My first protector and cohost, Sophia, is in charge. She is what we call the System Over Watcher. She's in charge of watching over me and the system. When I was younger I found it difficult that an alter held more power than I did since it was my body. Now I realize that she holds more power to protect me and everyone inside. Second in command is Caton. Sometimes Sophia needs to take a break in the system; she'll go to a little hut built specifically for her and Ashton when they need to handle personal business. Caton takes over then, and deals with everything while Sophia is gone. It's not technically a hierarchy, but some consider it that way.

*

SUNSHINE PURCELL
Denise was diagnosed with 17
personalities in 1995 at age 30

I hold the power, kind of. I don't tell them what to do. I may write and ask, or have someone ask them. But I find that the younger the alter, the more powerful they might be, and act out. I figured out that more traumatic incidents happened at a young age, and concerned a child, or in some cases a baby, or toddler. They are very powerful but are also the most loving. They just want to be treated like any children, teens, and people do. They eat and speak and have talents. I know there are a few who will voice concerns about the others, or about health, depression, isolation, or triggers. So whoever is out has the power.

*

ERICKA REEVE
Ericka was diagnosed with over 25
personalities in 2013 at age 26

The alter named A seems to have been the boss for a long time, in a way, but not fully. She just tends to be the loudest, and most in your face when needed. I struggle with them all for many different reasons. They all hold a certain amount of power. This depends entirely on the situation and the people who are around.

*

CHRIS ROBIN
Chris was diagnosed with at least
7 personalities in 2013 at age 49

I became used to having the parts of me take over when I was not able to deal with situations. There is one part of me that is much more aggressive and bossy, and can be a bully. All my parts know how to stay clear of that part, and not get in that part's way. I don't know that I would say there's a hierarchy or chain of command. For me, it doesn't feel like that. For the most part, I think the group dynamics are such that everyone knows they have strengths and weaknesses and have figured out how to interact and interject themselves when needed. When there is a disagreement or struggle for control, I have learned to lock them away in their rooms for a time. Again, I am beginning to realize and learn that this is not the healthiest way to deal with the parts of me, and until I process what is going on with that part of me, that part is going to continue to disrupt my inner world and eventually my outer world. I am learning how to have more compassion and understanding for all the parts, and find a way to have everyone work together. It's a process, not an event, so I am continuing to learn and heal.

*

QUINN ROSE
Quinn was diagnosed with 9
personalities in 2016 at age 21

I don't hold any power. My alter Raven controls the alters.

*

AYA SAKURA
Aya has been living with 7
personalities since childhood

We used to have a system head for quite a while. This was Makah (with the help of Sabrina) at first, and later on Sayu, and after that Lucy. The job of that system head was mainly planning who was doing what, and when, making rules, keeping everyone up to date, and getting everyone out at the right time, and in again. Other jobs that the system head had were, for example, making sure none of our belongings got lost and checking if everyone did their job. Makah also made strategic decisions for the whole system and kept everyone in check. The main reason that Makah got help from Sabrina is because Makah could not talk to everyone in the system. Sabrina had contact with a few others whom Makah could not talk to, so with having Sabrina to help her, Makah could get orders and messages through the whole system.

After Makah and Sabrina integrated (they became Sayu), Sayu took over the position and the duties as system head. She rarely came out and mostly helped out and managed everything from the background. At some point she stepped back and disappeared. I say disappeared because she's either integrated or hiding, I don't know which. This is when Lucy took over part of the role of system head. Lucy wasn't powerful enough to initiate a switch and get alters in and out like Makah and Sayu used to be able to do, so Lucy just planned everything, kept everyone up to date. Lucy also made sure to keep track of how everyone felt, and helped me pick a university and a bachelor's program. After half a year, she also disappeared (again, I don't know what became of her), because I stopped studying and going to work. At this point three of us were left: me, Brianna, and Clive. None of us is very suitable for a job as system head, so now we are kind of freestyling it, but it is not like everyone does what others say. Clive honors my wishes as well as Brianna's, but that does not stop him from smoking while I and Brianna wish he wouldn't. Brianna listens only to her husband, Clive, but mainly does whatever she wants. I just try to do my best and make everyone happy. I make all the most important decisions, with the support of both Clive and Brianna. Together with Clive, I try to plan everything so we can get through the week as smoothly as possible. We use an electronic calendar, which really helps a lot. The three of us make rules together as we go and try to function on a base of trust and respect.

At this point Clive is the one who comes closest to a system head. He knows the most about our system, and really likes to figure out all sorts of things about our system, which is why he knows so much. He also is the calmest, the oldest, and acts the most mature. We all take responsibility for our actions. If Brianna causes trouble, I and Clive also apologise and help to clean up the mess. We have always functioned this way, since Makah thought this would be the best way to avoid trouble.

*

FLOSS SCOTT
Floss was diagnosed with at least
4 personalities in 2016 at age 48

Out of all my alters I would say that Miss Protector comes out a lot when I'm vulnerable, hurt, upset or need protecting. She stays until she feels I can cope again. She will switch in and out when I don't have control, and she protects me. When I get upset or stressed I will conk out, and that will be followed by a seizure and then my alter Little Me will appear for a while until I conk out again. Miss Protector will then appear for days or weeks before she allows my host back. So overall Miss Protector is probably the most powerful one of them all.

*

PAULA SUNDWALL
Paula was diagnosed with dissociative amnesia in 2006 at age
36 and diagnosed with at least 4 personalities in 2014 at age 44

It might seem that I am in charge because I am out so much of the time, and because there seems to be some fear of me by the alters who all remain quiet and withdrawn. But I feel that there is one stronger alter who is really the leader. I think of her as an assertive and aggressive woman, and have tentatively named her Jordan, though I don't know why. I think that although Jordan gets me into trouble sometimes, overall she protects all of us, keeps things organized, keeps the harmful ones in as much as possible, and stands up for me when I won't do it for myself.

*

KERRYJANE VOTH
Kerryjane was diagnosed with
35 alters in 2013 at age 53

Through the last three years of trauma therapy, it has become abundantly apparent that there is not one host or director. I have been able to develop a co-consciousness with an observer who is able to help give an overview of some alters, access to memories among alters, an interpreter that can speak for alters, and have a stronger sense of love and caring and empathy for the system as a whole. It's only when all these alters are working together that we are able to get the best cooperation between us, and the system as a whole. This collective must be very careful that they don't come off as bossy or un-empathetic, or the system will shut down and lose cooperation.

*

Beneath
BY SUNSHINE

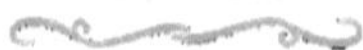

Look into my eyes and tell me what you see

The things I lack the most are the things that can set me free

Toss away my emotions don't bother with me anymore

The reflection I see in the mirror is the face I choose to ignore.

What lies beneath it all is pure and simple pain

waiting to be awoken from all that still remain.

Pulling away the layers, bit by bit and piece by piece

What lies beneath the surface so much still to release.

Look deep into my soul, all tattered and all torn

Lacking the ability of letting myself just mourn

Entangled webs of deceit never to be known

Forever seeming uncertain and forever feeling alone.

Look into my heart entangled in chains that bind

Searching for that forever love that seems impossible to find

My spirit has been broken to afraid again to fight

Hold for me a candle that guides me to the light.

What is, what will be, forever uncertainty

To cry, to scream, clawing at the wall

Where it hides, where it bleeds,

what lies beneath it all.

CHAPTER ELEVEN

Living with Triggers

Ideas come from somewhere. People don't come up with these ideas from nowhere. Something triggers your thoughts. -LAZARO HERNANDEZ

Triggers are sensory stimuli such as sights, sounds, and smells associated with a particular trauma, and dissociation is an overload response. Do you and your alters all share the same triggers? How do you manage or cope with triggers when they occur?

*

ADRIANNE ALLEN-LANG
Adrianne was diagnosed with 10
personalities in 2015 at age 18

We all share basically the same triggers. Things being thrown, shouting, violence, abandonment, sleeping alone, being touched in a certain spot on our back, large crowds of strangers. We're pretty good these days with dealing with triggering situations without having meltdowns, but we all still get extreme anxiety from having to go through them.

*

GAIL BUSWELL
Gail was diagnosed with 13
personalities in 2002 at age 24

We seem to be triggered by everything and everyone at the moment. We find it very difficult to verbalize what causes us to trigger, so we tend to internalize our fears which causes extreme levels of anxiety. We use blowing bubbles as an effective way to ground ourselves and control our breathing while triggered. Life hasn't always been this way, and I hope things settle down soon.

*

KATT HART
Katt was diagnosed with hundreds
of personalities in 2011 at age 20

We have quite a lot of triggers, some that seem quite odd to people, and some that are more widely accepted. We struggle very much with details of abuse. While a lot of our abuse memories are cut off from a lot of us, the triggers still really affect the ones who are aware of it. Sexual abuse details, sometimes even minor mentions, can be absolutely huge triggers for us. They typically either trigger out alters who are completely sex-repulsed or sex-phobic, or on the opposite side can trigger alters who are very sexual and will try to have sex with as many people as they can.

Most of us are triggered by medical situations. Just going to see a general practitioner is terrifying and brings up horrible memories and feelings. Unfortunately, this leaves us avoiding medical things as much as we're able to, which could be very damaging to our health.

We have some odd triggers that are related to popular movies and books, ones where we don't often bring up the details but are unfortunately some of the most common triggers we come across, since they are very popular. These movies and books were either used during the abuse or were around in one way or another when we were being abused. This has resulted in alters who are based on fictional characters. That's a huge thing that we're scared of, people knowing, in case people then assume we're faking it. These alters are usually the main ones triggered when those movies or books are brought up, or if there's imagery or quotes from them.

We have triggers related to certain video games as well, thanks to abusive exes, and video games that were played during bad times in childhood. There are so many more triggers, but just thinking about what they are can be really hard and upsetting. Sometimes, groups of alters are triggered by certain things. This can make it really difficult when those triggers come up, because we can end up rapidly switching between the ones who are triggered, or with other alters trying desperately to hold them back if it could somehow result in harm to us or someone else. It's horrible, and often the more alters who are triggered, the harder it is to gain back control or hold back switching.

If just one alter is triggered, then another alter who isn't triggered can usually step forward or stay out while other alters calm down the one who's triggered. We keep distractions with us while we're outside. Inside the house, we have a lot of positive things to focus on instead of the triggers, so if we do get triggered, we try very hard to use these things. Usually they're things like stuffed toys, a book to write in, games on our phone, animated movies, toys, putty, and glitter jars. These sorts of things can help, depending on how bad the trigger is and how many alters are affected. One of the most helpful things we've found is using things like bath bombs, as long as the trigger isn't body-related. We get a bath bomb and watch it fizz and make colors. It's even better if the water will go glittery, as it gives us another thing to focus on.

*

AMELIA JOUBERT
Amelia was diagnosed with 12
personalities in 2013 at age 15

One of my biggest triggers is the "Alice In Wonderland" movie, though I have no idea why. I can't watch the movie at all, and pictures and quotes from it make me very uncomfortable. Another big trigger of mine is conflict. I tend to get stressed out by serious conversations, and it either makes me dissociate or sends me into a panic attack. My little who holds trauma, Aliya, is triggered by loud noises and is very scared of anything unfamiliar. We have a necklace with many things on it. I call it our grounding necklace. Each thing on the necklace is important to one or several of us, and it helps us stay safe.

*

AMANDA LINEBACK
Amanda was diagnosed with hundreds
of personalities in 2013 at age 31

My triggers have changed over time. Almost everything in life was a trigger for a while. I am not sure who the triggers belong to, but here are some of the things that are highly triggering for us: trains, ice cream trucks, box cutters, and doorbells. I was just made to switch, so I can't talk about this anymore. I am getting too close to something that is not supposed to be shared, and now I can't feel my body.

*

JANE MACDONALD
Jane was diagnosed with 3 personalities in
2014 at age 35, and currently has 6 alters

I have a difficult time knowing what triggers me and my alters, as I am only occasionally co-conscious with them. I know that I share many triggers with my youngest alter, Clara. We are both extremely hypervigilant due to anxiety disorders. We are easily triggered by loud, sudden noises such as arguing, traffic, banging, and sometimes thunder. We both share a fear of men who are tall, thin, and balding. I have a feeling this is related to the ongoing abuse I suffered at the hands of a male relative throughout childhood, adolescence and even into adulthood. This is a problematic trigger as this is what my psychiatrist looks like.

Not all of my alters share the same triggers. To complicate things further, some things, such as certain types of music, which calm down one alter, usually Clara, can trigger a different alter. This makes it very difficult to cope. For example, I will play certain types of music because it is one of the few things that calm Clara down, but by doing so I risk triggering Angela, who becomes very angry and aggressive. Music can also be a trigger for me and Clara, particularly when it has themes of domestic violence or aggression, such as Lady Gaga's new song "Til It Happens To You." Sometimes I like listening to this song, because it reminds me that I am not alone, but other times it is too triggering and can cause Clara to come out and curl into a ball and cry or hide under the covers on the bed. I am not aware of the triggers of the other alters, because I do not know them as well, and am usually less co-conscious with them than I am with Clara.

I have had great difficulty in trying to cope with triggers. For Clara, my youngest alter, I try to make a safe space for her to go to, with stuffed animals and soft blankets and pillows. For myself it is more difficult. I have noise-reducing headphones to wear when the construction noise coming from the new building next door gets to be too much, or the arguing and banging in the unit below me. When I am out in public, I can't wear the headphones and have to find other ways to deal with my distress. I have tried to learn meditation and grounding techniques, but find I can't always remember them or don't find them useful. Up until recently this sensitivity to noise was a serious issue, as my psychiatrist works in a rather noisy environment. However, he is willing to see me during less busy times and at a less busy location in order to work with me and prevent me from completely dissociating during our sessions. He has been very accommodating toward this trigger, but most life circumstances cannot be modified this way. I can't get rid of all the traffic or construction in my city, for example. All I can do is try to get away from the triggers, or use the grounding techniques that I've learned over the years and hope that they work. This fear of being triggered when outside or in public is a large reason for my isolation and extreme reluctance to leave my apartment. At home, and with my psychiatrist, I can have some control over things. Out in the larger world, I do not have control.

*

CRYSTALIE MATULEWICZ
Crystalie was diagnosed with dissociative
identity disorder in 2015 at age 29

When you endure twenty-nine years of abuse, you end up with a lot of triggers. Over time, I've learned to manage some of them, and they don't affect me nearly as badly as they used to. Some triggers have not been so easy to manage.

My parts and I have a lot of food triggers. Food was often used as a tool for manipulation, and was taken away as a form of punishment. As a result, I developed a lot of food-related issues and triggers. Even though I am in a different environment now, I still experience situations that remind me of what happened in the past. My parts and I carry a lot of shame and guilt about eating. The smallest thing that seems insignificant to most can feel devastating to us. Someone eating our food, or someone offering us food, can trigger bad memories and unhealthy behaviors like starvation.

Certain words are triggers for me, words that were used against me in childhood. Even though I have always excelled academically, my mother often called me dumb and stupid. Derogatory names are also a trigger because they are reminders of past verbal abuse. I have difficulty fighting back or asserting my needs when someone uses those words against me. I couldn't stand up against my mother, and even when it's someone else doing the name-calling, I shut down just like I did before. I internalize those names, believing that they are true. This often leads to self-hatred and self-harm behavior if I can't work through it right away.

Emotions are a trigger for several parts and me. I have a lot of body memories connected to certain feelings. I get really bad headaches when I am depressed. Feeling depressed is a trigger for me because of the experience I had as a teenager. I have trouble admitting when I am feeling that way, because I still fear being punished for it like I was when I was younger. Anger tends to trigger dissociation, and is one of my most complicated emotions.

One of my biggest triggers, which fortunately hasn't been as much of an issue now that I ran away, is when someone compares me to my mother. Many people believe that I look physically similar to my mother. It didn't help that my mother would wear my clothes and dye her hair the same color as mine, which I believe she did because she knew it triggered me. Whenever a coworker or acquaintance of my mother's would comment about how much I was just like my mother, it would make me physically ill to the point of vomiting. In my mind, when they were saying I was just like my mother, then I believed I must be like her in every way. I knew she was a child abuser, so that meant I must be one too. It made me hate myself in ways I could never describe out loud.

Showers are a bad trigger for both my parts and me, as that is one of the places where we were abused. It's not as triggering as it has been in the past, but the experience is still very anxiety-provoking. It's difficult, because showers are a necessary part of self-care, so I can't just avoid it like I can with other triggers. To work through the anxiety, I take extra precautions to ensure safety. I always lock the door. I check behind the shower curtain before I turn on the water. I keep saying "I am safe, we are safe" over and over until I'm done. Sometimes I do end up dissociating. I come back wondering why the shower water is cold and realize that I've been in there a lot longer than I intended to. It has definitely been one of my most difficult triggers to work through.

Specific dates are triggers, because they are reminders of really traumatic experiences. Mother's Day is one. On that day and in the weeks before the holiday each year, I am bombarded with images of loving mothers, and commands to "love your mother because she's the only one you'll ever have." Being a narcissist, my mother treated the holiday like it was her birthright. Even though I am away from her now, the day is a reminder of all the things my mother was not for me; she was a mother only for my birth, and nothing more than that. She was my abuser, and having a day to honor all the hurt she put me through creates a rage in me that is difficult to suppress. My parts have a hard time with it, too. They don't understand why we didn't have a mother like they see everywhere around us.

April 25 is the most difficult anniversary date trigger for me. That is the date on which I attempted suicide. It wasn't the attempt itself that has made it so difficult, but the way my family reacted. In a moment of desperation, while I was physically ill, bruised all over my body, and unable to hear, I told my family what I had done. Instead of being concerned, they took away my phone, leaving me unable to call for help, and went about their day like nothing had happened. I could have died. I should have died. And my family didn't care. It hurt me in a way I can't describe. I lost my family. I lost what little bit I had left of my heart. I lost all hope that day. Every year when April approaches, I start getting flashbacks and start to hurt the same way I did then, and end in a deep depression. I've attempted suicide twice on that date since. It's an annual reminder of the tremendous pain I experienced that day.

There are so many other triggers that I just can't explain thoroughly in a few paragraphs, and they are triggers we encounter regularly. My main method of minimizing triggers is to avoid them, but some things just can't be avoided. Knocking on doors is a trigger for several of my parts and me. It induces tremendous panic and flashbacks. I have missed meetings and angered people because I couldn't handle knocking on a door. Instead, I just run away or go off crying.

I try to engage in positive self-talk to counteract the negative judgments that tend to accompany a trigger, but sometimes that doesn't work. Distraction is a useful tool. I carry around a safe book to read, a coloring book, and clay in case I experience a trigger and need to do something self-soothing. I wear bracelets to remind us that we are safe, that we are free, that it's okay to feel, and that we can ask for help. Writing also helps, and the feedback I get from others often helps me work through the triggering experiences. I go to therapy a couple of times a week, so I work through triggers there as well. There are lots of ways I can cope with triggers. The difficulty is actually utilizing the methods when I need to, instead of getting caught in the experience.

*

ALICIA PETTIS
Alicia was diagnosed with 40
personalities in 2015 at age 16

Some of my triggers are very simple, such as a towel, and some are very complex, such as being touched in my sleep. The towel stems from my father constantly beating me and breaking my nose. He would throw a towel in my face and tell me to clean it up. The touching stems from very recent abuse that I escaped from. I can barely speak of this trigger because it's such a fresh wound, but there are exceptions to it. If I'm sleeping with someone and I know that person is there, touching won't affect me. But if they walk into my room and touch me when I'm sleeping, I jolt awake and have a panic attack.

I don't share a lot of triggers with my alters, mainly because they hold the memories for me, so the trigger may affect me slightly, but not enough. It's as if I sense déja vu, but on a very different scale than the alter. I'll understand that it's triggering somehow, but it won't make me scared or panic like my own triggers do. When either of us is triggered, we're brought into the system and either play with Lyn, go for a walk in the woods, or play on the playground. If I'm triggered beyond any of those options, I'm sent to a place we call the Dark Room. It's similar to a void; I can't hear, see, or speak from this room, and I can calm down in peace and quiet. Sometimes Stella will join me in the Dark Room and project stars all around, so it seems like I'm surrounded by stars and nebulae.

*

SUNSHINE PURCELL
Denise was diagnosed with 17
personalities in 1995 at age 30

I am triggered by smells, hands, grandfathers, lilac smell, and television shows that portray abuse similar to what I've been through; these are some of the triggers I know of. When an alter feels a trigger, he or she will come out and cry and scream until it subsides. As for lilac season, we all can sense that the season is approaching before blooming begins; it's like a sixth sense. It starts with flashbacks and nightmares, we're afraid to sleep, and life becomes even more exhausting for all. It stays this way until the flowers die, and then it subsides. It's the biggest trigger that is outwardly known and felt by all. The little ones hold that trigger, but all of us can feel it. It's like layers upon layers of random thoughts, fear of everything, crying spells, and depression. The other triggers are on the dates that they happened. That much I've worked out in therapy, like the dates of my rape, when I was taken hostage, and abuse by an ex-husband. They are felt by the alter who took them. I feel a higher sense of alert and awareness but that's because I'm the main host.

*

ERICKA REEVE
Ericka was diagnosed with over
25 personalities in 2013 at age 26

We do not all share the same triggers, which in a way surprises me. I now know and understand far more while we've been in therapy, this year especially.

One of my parts helps literally everyone. She helps me now that I know of her and what she does and is capable of. When we're triggered or I am triggered, she'll begin by trying to have me focus on something in the room, and then she'll rub my back, legs or arms. With the help of another, they can almost reboot all my senses in a way. All of a sudden there is just nothing, and then they gradually bring me back from that. It's frightening at times, but now I know what's going on, and I do find it easier to refocus and become more present when they do that, as opposed to pulling myself or others away from something triggering.

Before, I would become uncomfortable and then get an angry sensation and not remember a thing. All I knew was that when I became angry, I blacked out. I now am aware it happened for many other reasons, but anger was what I had personally noticed.

So many things are triggering that it literally can be anything or everything. There are varying degrees for all of us. For myself, I find that certain smells are far more triggering than anything else.

*

CHRIS ROBIN
Chris was diagnosed with at least
7 personalities in 2013 at age 49

I am still relatively new at this DID stuff, so I am just now learning to identify when I dissociate and have to really work hard to find out what triggered it when this happens. Most of the time close friends or my therapist have to show me or explain to me what triggered a switch.

I do know that my triggers come in various fashions: sounds, smells, places, phrases, or even thoughts or memories. I think many of my parts have shared some of the same triggers, but then sometimes only certain parts react to the triggers. Mostly I find that the triggers take me outside my window of tolerance, and it becomes very difficult to either get the other parts of me to help out, or reach out for help. It's hard to even remember the things I've been taught to help ground myself back to the present, because I also suffer from complicated grief and PTSD along with depression. So my brain has become very good at switching, and my parts know when I can't cope with a situation and just take over.

The problem is that in order to live in this unforgiving world, I have to understand that I will be triggered and I have to learn how to deal with the symptoms and find ways to hide them from the public, which can be very lonely and isolating. Retreating to the privacy of my car, or slipping away into a restroom or another room, or even just going home are the coping strategies that I now use when triggered. I also have been able to notice when it is happening and find time later, when I am alone, to begin to process the event and figure out what the trigger was. I now have some skills in my toolbox to help with the emotions and get me grounded back to the present. Sometimes I spend many moments wondering if locking myself away from the world and away from the possibility of being triggered might be a healthier life for me. But the obligations and need for involvement in the world forces me to learn to face the world.

*
QUINN ROSE
Quinn was diagnosed with 9
personalities in 2016 at age 21

High stress, drinking, a lookalike to an ex, these are the only ones I'm aware of so far. And I don't know how to cope. I come to the next day or so and just go about my daily life again. I try not to think about it too hard.

*

AYA SAKURA
Aya has been living with 7
personalities since childhood

We do not all have the same triggers. Quite the opposite, actually. We each have specific triggers. The triggers are related to the job my alters have in the system. There are a whole lot of triggers I could write down, but I'm only comfortable with writing about more neutral triggers, so I'm doing that.

One of Brianna's triggers we are comfortable writing about is places with a lot of people around, especially if I have to interact with people. I am very introverted, but Brianna is extremely extroverted. She loves to interact with people and go to parties and events like that. She gets energy off it, while I am drained at some point.

A trigger for Clive is when my body is sick or not too well. He's very good at sensing what's wrong and takes care of it. He also comes out when I'm very tired. He doesn't take very much energy, which enables him to get through the day when I'm running low on energy and falling asleep. Both of them are triggered when I'm anxious or stressed. They both cope differently. Clive copes short-term with stress by breathing very slowly and forcing himself to act very relaxed, a kind of fake-it-until-you-make-it, and when he's got the chance he smokes. In the long term he tries manage the system so that stress and anxiety are reduced to a minimum. Brianna copes with anxiety by drinking alcohol and recently also by meditating.

*

FLOSS SCOTT
Floss was diagnosed with at least
4 personalities in 2016 at age 48

I find that two of the biggest triggers are mess and people taking advantage of me. This will trigger Miss Protector and she can be very nasty if she has to be. These are some of my triggers: seizures, conking out, blackouts, stress, upset, trauma, mess, laziness, someone not listening, lying, stealing from me, taking advantage of me, rejection, and bullying. These are just a few of my triggers and they can bring out the nasty in Miss Protector.

*

KERRYJANE VOTH
Kerryjane was diagnosed with
35 alters in 2013 at age 53

I have a few triggers that I'm comfortable talking about. If anyone, including myself, gets angry, it is a really strong trigger to shut down. This trigger was trained into me as a very young child by my caregivers. Anger was not allowed under any circumstances. I was told over and over again that to be angry was to "release fifty-two different poisons into my body and I would surely die."

Triangulation: When two or more people join me to socialize, I become very nervous, because I was raised by a narcissistic caregiver who pitted family members against each other. I'm much more comfortable socializing one-on-one.

Money is triggering because it is a form of control. I am not motivated by money, because then I would be controlled by whoever was paying me.

*

If
BY SUNSHINE

If only if only I could go in and reach you, a little girl about ten,
I'd scoop you up and hug you, protecting you from back then,
wiping away tears from those beautiful green eyes,
kissing all your hurt away, shielding you from all those lies.

If I could go in a reach you a young girl about fifteen,
I'd take you by the hand guiding you through the unforeseen,
lift your shameful head and tell you you're not bad.
There's strength in who you are, so please don't look so sad.

If I could go in and reach you, a young woman in despair,
I'd take away the pain he caused, so far beyond repair.
I'd mend your broken spirit and send you on your way,
to smile again with the rising sun, gladly facing a brand new day.

If I could go in and reach you, a woman who has felt
nothing but abuse and fear, searching to be free,
I'd pick you up and take you to a place that's safe to be;
showing you there is still love in places you've yet to see.

If I could go in and reach you, a woman far beyond her years,
I'd warm you with my love and dry up all your tears.
I'd tell you to be proud and never scared of who you are,
for time can ease the memories and love can hide the scars.

If I could go in and reach you all,
oh what a place this world would be!
For every single one of you equal all of me.
I try to go in and reach you but I can't, you're too far away,
so I dream of when we'll all be together,
maybe some other way.

CHAPTER TWELVE

Living with Physical Pain

We live in bodies that are fearfully and wonderfully
made, yet they are not immune to illness and pain.
-ADAM HAMILTON

Physical pain can provoke severe anxiety and be a powerful trigger to dissociate. How do you handle physical discomfort or pain resulting from everyday life, like medical exams?

*

ADRIANNE ALLEN-LANG
Adrianne was diagnosed with 10
personalities in 2015 at age 18

We have zero issues with physical pain (ha ha). Nurse, one in our system, is the keeper and dealer of pain, so she takes seventy-five percent of all pain so we don't experience it.

*

GAIL BUSWELL
Gail was diagnosed with 13
personalities in 2002 at age 24

Pain causes us to dissociate. One of my others is programmed to endure pain and will come forward at times of planned painful procedures like blood draws and invasive medical procedures. I suffer from fibromyalgia, so I am in chronic physical pain daily. None of the others share this pain with me.

*

KATT HART
Katt was diagnosed with hundreds
of personalities in 2011 at age 20

We often avoid a lot of things that would cause us physical pain, especially anything medical, due to the intense triggers surrounding that sort of thing. On the other hand, some of us are absolutely obsessed with tattoos and piercings. Some of us will avoid those things and be scared, though. One of our alters loves piercings, so he got our lip and septum pierced, but another alter was scared and nearly left before they started. I have a feeling that others who are like that alter will keep adding more piercings and tattoos when money is available and the opportunity presents itself.

*

AMELIA JOUBERT
Amelia was diagnosed with 12
personalities in 2013 at age 15

Pain makes me dissociate. When it's pain we know is coming, like getting a shot or our blood drawn, my alter Jax will come out and take the pain. I also get ovarian cysts which can be very painful and sometimes trigger a switch while other times just send me into a dissociated state I call drifting. We plan on getting our first tattoo early next year and Jax has already agreed to be out for it.

*

AMANDA LINEBACK
Amanda was diagnosed with hundreds
of personalities in 2013 at age 31

Pain does not bother me at all. I can make myself not feel anything. I have learned to completely turn it off physically. I have never avoided activities because I was scared of pain.

*

JANE MACDONALD
Jane was diagnosed with 3 personalities in
2014 at age 35, and currently has 6 alters

I consider myself very fortunate in this respect, as I do not have to deal with much physical pain. That being said, when I do experience pain it tends to trigger some of my alters, particularly my youngest alter. I don't know entirely how she reacts, as I am not usually co-conscious with her, but I do know that if I am having stomach pain in particular, she tends to come out and curl up into a ball, usually on my bed, hides under the covers and starts to cry. I know this because I'll wake in this position or because I can feel her coming out and am briefly aware before she takes over.

Since I am unaware of how other alters handle pain, I do my best to avoid things that might be painful, such as donating blood or getting bloodwork, or physical exams by my doctor. I've recently started to get weekly allergy shots at my doctor's office to treat severe allergies, but fortunately this hasn't seemed to trigger any alters.

*

CRYSTALIE MATULEWICZ
Crystalie was diagnosed with dissociative
identity disorder in 2015 at age 29

My parts and I have an interesting relationship with pain. When I am fully present I can experience pain, but there are times when my pain tolerance can either be very high or very low because my parts experience pain differently. Some parts experience pain intensely, more so than normal. If I know ahead of time that something is going to be painful, I let my parts know what is going to happen, so they don't get scared and it doesn't get chaotic. That way, the parts who are scared of pain can find a safe place.

Some of my parts were created to not feel pain as a result of the abuse we experienced when younger. Some people think the ability to not feel pain is good, and in some ways it is. I suffer from physical conditions that cause regular pain, and sometimes it is overwhelming. On the other hand, pain has a purpose; it tells you when something is wrong. If you're not able to feel pain, you're not going to know when something is awry. This is the downside. I've broken my foot before and walked on it because I didn't feel the pain until later. The damage got worse, even though I felt nothing at all. I've been hospitalized several times with pneumonia because I didn't experience the physical pain until it got to the point where I couldn't breathe on my own. I once burned my abdomen leaning over the stove. I didn't realize the burner was on until I smelled something burning. By that time, it had already burned through my shirt and most of my skin. I couldn't feel the pain at all.

I can't really change the way I or my parts experience pain, so I have to manage in other ways. I try to be aware of the physical changes in my body. I know that if my hands are blue, I need to focus on my breathing. I keep track of bumps and bruises. I try to ground myself so I can be more aware of what is going on, not only on the outside, but inside my body as well. I try to go to doctors to keep medical issues in check. Overall, it's not so much the fear of physical pain that concerns me the most. It's the fear of not being able to feel pain at all that proves to be the most troublesome.

*

ALICIA PETTIS
Alicia was diagnosed with 40
personalities in 2015 at age 16

Doctors scare me, as do hospitals and any authority figure. When it comes to an exam or check-up, I'm either not present or desensitized from the entire thing. Cas is an alter who, when co-conscious with me, makes me feel numb toward everything. He'll step in when I stay in control but am scared. As for donating blood or getting tattoos, I'm not scared of either. I am scared of needles but I realize that if it's my choice and I really want to do it, then it doesn't faze me for long.

*

SUNSHINE PURCELL
Denise was diagnosed with 17
personalities in 1995 at age 30

For me, the only anxiety I have is gynecologic exams because those were the parts hurt most often. They feel cut off from my body. I get very scared if I need to have a test. I can't, in any way possible, have a male doctor. As for any other fear of pain, I have been able to turn my senses off. I can handle it with very little discomfort. That's the way my mind handles it. I went through the pain of cigars being burned into my inner thighs, so it was a mind game with the abuser. I could never give in and let him win, even if it meant my own demise.

*

ERICKA REEVE
Ericka was diagnosed with over 25
personalities in 2013 at age 26

I handle this well, or so I thought. When I was young, doctors thought I had that rare genetic disorder where you're incapable of feeling pain sensations properly. After even testing in adulthood, that is partially true, but not the specific condition they meant. I have a milder form.

When I was younger, my parts just cut off the pain or took it themselves so I didn't feel it. This still occurs from time to time, but they will just come in fully and handle it themselves. We're working on it now and things are getting better, which is paradoxical I suppose, because I do have a few physical conditions that exacerbate pain but combine with the other physical conditions, and then it's manageable. I don't recall ever crying from pain. An example from my childhood: I had broken my arm from stepping out of the shower and had no idea until nearly two weeks later when it just didn't move. I began my own research into what could cause that. I never did stumble across DID (which was called multiple personalities at that point) but I am aware now that it's a contributing factor in addition to the DID.

*

CHRIS ROBIN
Chris was diagnosed with at least
7 personalities in 2013 at age 49

I have always known that I hate when people touch or examine me, either physically or mentally. So I've managed to spend most of my life relatively healthy, and I don't see doctors very regularly. After watching my partner get poked and prodded and undergo cancer treatment, I now have a phobia of doctors and hospitals.

I can tune out pain when I have to, and I can tolerate more pain than most people. I used to think that I was really just a big wimp, but when pushed into needing help for physical pain, I find myself medicating with both over-the-counter drugs and illegal and legal drugs, and going to see a doctor only in extreme cases. When my partner was with me, I could tolerate doctors and physical pain more. Now knowing I have DID, I realize that there are parts of me who have contained the physical and emotional pains of my life, and I need to give them some relief. Sometimes I almost enjoy physical pain just to feel something, because I think sometimes I just overcompensate or ignore the pain, cover it up or avoid it and feel nothing at all. I also have to learn that feelings, both physical and emotional, are normal.

*

QUINN ROSE
Quinn was diagnosed with 9
personalities in 2016 at age 21

Every so often an alter will come out due to physical pain from pinched nerves, or if I accidentally get hit. I do fear the needle prick from testing my blood sugar due to one bruising my finger, and I know I black out when they try.

*

AYA SAKURA
Aya has been living with 7
personalities since childhood

Luckily, we are blessed with a healthy body, so we don't need regular doctor exams. I can handle most of my aches and pains myself. But I am a female and have a female body, so I experience periods and the cramps that go with it. The first twenty-four hours are the worst, and cause me to dissociate very much. Sometimes it's so bad that it triggers out Clive, who handles all the physical things and has a higher pain tolerance. He takes painkillers for it. When I burned my hand while cooking, Clive came out and took care of both my burn and the food. Headaches also are a trigger for Clive, if they are bad enough. He then does whatever he thinks is best to help relieve the headache. If I get a moderate headache, it causes me to dissociate. Unfortunately, painkillers can't take my headache pain away. Brianna absolutely hates pain in any form so if she hurts herself, she goes back in immediately. Clive then comes out and takes care of it. We do donate blood, but that doesn't really cause pain. Brianna faints at the sight of blood, so I'll only give blood if I'm completely sure she's not around.

*

FLOSS SCOTT
Floss was diagnosed with at least
4 personalities in 2016 at age 48

I suffer from centralization of the nervous system and chronic pain disorder with pain from the neck down to the lower back. However, ever since I was a young girl, I hated and couldn't handle needles, so I had a fear of blood tests and other injections. I once almost kicked a doctor across the ward when they were trying to fit a drip into me. In the end, they held me down while I was kicking and screaming. Even at the dentist's, they had to put me to sleep before they could perform a filling as I couldn't handle the needle when they tried to numb the gums. I could never have a tattoo or administer needles into my body. I hated them when I was growing up, and still have that fear and hate now.

*

KERRYJANE VOTH
Kerryjane was diagnosed with
35 alters in 2013 at age 53

I still dissociate quite a bit. It is an everyday occurrence. I will switch alters as well. My service dog will help distract me, and will distract others from giving me any unwanted attention. I do a lot of comfort talking to all the alters. I hold long conversations where we explore all the concerns and find as much educational information as possible to give the system a heads-up beforehand. Leaving less to the imagination is the best way to deal with the anticipation of pain. When it comes to dealing with the pain itself, I have a very high tolerance. Usually deep breathing is sufficient to be able to manage it, and if not, then I switch to an alter who can tolerate it. If the pain persists, then dissociation takes over and I don't remember anything.

*

Beginnings
BY SUNSHINE

I'm beginning to remember

that's buried oh so deep

always there awaiting me

in forever restless sleep

I'm beginning to feel

the utmost pain

only slivers of my innocence

are all that still remain.

I'm beginning to hear the truth

I wish to ignore

as every memory that bound me

opens a new door.

I'm beginning to cry

at the love that I lost

the price I've had to pay,

no matter was the cost.

I'm beginning to remember

all that's buried oh so deep

I'm beginning to remember,

but its only in my sleep.

*

CHAPTER THIRTEEN

Struggling with Self Harm

A writer's main tool is his memory—his own memory, the collective memory of his people. And the strongest memory is the one that is created by a wound to the heart. -ANATOLY RYBAKOV

Some individuals self-injure to temporarily relieve emotional pain. By inflicting harm, the brain releases calming hormones like dopamine and serotonin. Did you or do you engage in self-harm?

*

ADRIANNE ALLEN-LANG
Adrianne was diagnosed with 10
personalities in 2015 at age 18

We haven't self-harmed in four years now.

*

GAIL BUSWELL
Gail was diagnosed with 13
personalities in 2002 at age 24

I have self-harmed for as long as I can remember. It started with jabbing my pencil into the top of my leg and scraping my ruler along my arm until it bled. I have little memory of my childhood, so I am unsure if my scars come from self-harm or from the abuse I suffered.

*

KATT HART
Katt was diagnosed with hundreds
of personalities in 2011 at age 20

While we don't self-harm in the more well-known ways like cutting or burning, a lot of us do pick, scratch, starve, and isolate ourselves as a form of punishment. It doesn't exactly provide comfort, and it actually scares us a lot that we do these things, but we can't seem to help it. It's more of a compulsion than an actual coping method at this point.

There are alters who will cut themselves in the inner world, but thankfully we've managed to prevent them from doing it on the body so far. It's hard to hold back the alters who want to self-harm more severely, and it's hard for us and our partner to keep them from doing that sort of thing. We're very glad that it's working so far, or at least most of us are.

The idea of self-harm becoming addictive is probably one of the scary parts. Knowing people who cut and others with DID who wake up to mystery cuts all over their arms and legs scares us, and we don't want to end up having to experience that. It upsets some that we can't let them start cutting, but we want to try our very best to avoid it. There are some alters who want to self-harm who engage in BDSM to satisfy their need for pain, but in a controlled environment. It's sometimes not ideal when there's bruising or minor cuts, but we'd much rather they did that with someone safe and trusted than cut with no supervision, to make sure it isn't too bad and no controlled environment to get them to stop.

*

AMELIA JOUBERT
Amelia was diagnosed with 12
personalities in 2013 at age 15

I used to self-harm as a coping behavior, as did a few of my alters. I'm not really sure why it made me feel better in the moment, but it did. After doing it I would go into a spaced-out state, but it was different from my normal dissociation. One of my alters who no longer comes out, Eli, would also hurt our body by carving his name into my arm, but never very deep. Another who also doesn't come out anymore, Regna, would cut with a lot of shallow cuts all over. She even cut my neck, which led to a hospitalization. I have been able to lock these alters deep in our mind through therapy work, and I no longer self-harm.

*

AMANDA LINEBACK
Amanda was diagnosed with hundreds
of personalities in 2013 at age 31

Until two years ago I used self-harm as my emotional release. I blocked out physical pain, but my emotions hurt me. I cut myself because I needed to turn my emotional pain into a type of pain I could handle. I still have urges to self-harm. I keep a rubber band on my wrist, and if I want to self-harm I pull that rubber band and let it snap down. It works, and it does hurt.

*

JANE MACDONALD
Jane was diagnosed with 3 personalities in
2014 at age 35, and currently has 6 alters

I started self-harming during my first year of high school as a way to cope with overwhelming emotions. It started out small, a few scratches with tabs off of pop cans. It was my best friend's idea at the time and I was rife with emotional turmoil at that age, as many teenagers are, so I immediately latched on to it. Over time the cutting got worse. I cut with different objects, sometimes metal, sometimes glass, whatever I could find. By the time I became aware of my DID and alter personalities I had been self-harming for two decades. It is such an ingrained coping mechanism that I am not really able to stop. It is a part of me. It is what I do to release all the turmoil inside me. Although I am aware that it can be upsetting for my littlest alter, and I do try my hardest not to do it, I often feel like I have no other venue to release what I am feeling. Also troubling and perhaps even more difficult is that one of my other alters engages in self-harm as well. When she does it, it's actually far worse. The cuts are deeper and take longer to heal.

I've never felt the physical pain associated with self-harm. Right from the beginning, I dissociate when engaged in this behavior, so pain was not something I was aware of. I don't know if it is the sight of the blood, the pain, or something else that is upsetting to my youngest alters. Unfortunately, I have yet to find another solution.

I'd like to say that cutting makes everything better, that it takes away the inner turmoil I feel at the time, and makes everything more bearable. And sometimes it does, but only for a minute. When I did it back in high school, it helped me achieve a catharsis that nothing else seemed to be able to do. It helped me deal with the overwhelming emotions I felt. Now, after doing it for two decades, it just doesn't have the same effect. Yet I still feel compelled to do it when I feel strong emotions or feel particularly overwhelmed. It has also come to take on a self-punitive aspect. If I am feeling guilty, I will do it to punish myself. It's not the pain that is the punishment, as I rarely feel that. It's more the subsequent shame of having to hide my arms even during the hottest of days because of the scars I have. It is the constant reminder of my own inability to manage my emotions in a more healthy and productive way.

What scares me most about self-harm is that it's no longer the helpful tool that it once was. Now it has become an ingrained coping mechanism, and an entirely unhealthy one at that. The emotional release is brief, if at all. Often I am filled with even more emotions afterward: sad that I can't find another way to handle things, guilty about doing it yet again, angry at myself for being so weak. It also scares me that when my other personality does it, she cuts deeper, draws more blood, and leaves darker and more noticeable scars. It scares me that I am not aware of when she does it, and I can't control it (or her). It scares me that I engage in this behavior even without the rewards it once offered. It also scares me that one day it might not be enough and that I might take it too far, and have even more dire consequences than scars on my arms.

*

CRYSTALIE MATULEWICZ
Crystalie was diagnosed with dissociative
identity disorder in 2015 at age 29

I started self-harming before I even knew what self-harm was. Around age six I started scratching the skin on my arms and legs. I would keep scratching until I ended up with raw patches that took weeks to heal. People assumed they were just bad rashes. I realized later on what was really going on. I continued to scratch at various times, even into my adolescence and adulthood. We still sometimes scratch, but not nearly as often as I did when I was younger.

Around the age of ten, I started physically beating myself up. I repeatedly banged my wrists against the wall, and ended up spraining my wrist a few times because of it. I hit myself repeatedly, hard enough to cause bruises. It was very much a learned behavior rather than any kind of emotional release. I was beaten any time I was deemed bad, so I started punishing myself for anything I believed I did wrong, in the same ways my parents had done.

Around that same age, I started cutting myself. I was still being abused, so I couldn't get away with much damage without notice. When I was finally allowed to bathe myself, my cutting increased. Once or twice turned into ten or twenty at a time. I wore long sleeves to hide the marks. My high school guidance counselor found out and called my parents. My mother started body-checking me, and forcing me to undress so she could check for injuries. It was traumatizing, and only made my self-harm worse. Instead of doing it less, I just learned to hide it better.

As an adult, I engaged in more dangerous forms of self-harm. When I was in my twenties I once became so angry that I stabbed myself in the abdomen several times with a knife, causing permanent scarring. I've engaged in head-banging, repeatedly hitting my head against the wall up to fifty times. Several times I became disoriented and lost consciousness. I've also burned myself, resulting in second- and third-degree burns, some of which were treated with hospitalization. I now have permanent scarring.

I've also used more acceptable forms of self-harm. In the past I abused drugs that allowed me to forget everything going on around me. It helped me bury the emotions I didn't want to feel. While I've been able to stay clean, it's still a struggle. When life gets chaotic, as my life often does, the urge to use comes right back. I've also smoked on and off for the last eleven years. While most don't see smoking as self-harm, it is for me because I have COPD. I continue to smoke because part of me knows that smoking is killing me, and it's an easy way to self-destruct without leaving marks.

A big reason why I started self-harming as a child, and still do as an adult, was because I was not allowed to express feelings and emotions. I was not allowed to talk about how I was feeling, When I did express them, I got in trouble. So I learned to express them in other ways, like through self-harm. I couldn't say "I'm angry," so I beat myself up and banged my head. I couldn't say "I'm depressed," so I cut myself. I couldn't say "I'm hopeless," so I stabbed myself, hoping it would kill me. Self-harm was the only way I knew how to emote, and the only way that felt safe.

It's hard to explain. Sometimes I do it because I'm so numb that I need to feel something. Sometimes it's because I'm in so much pain inside and need something on the outside to make the inside pain feel valid. I can't explain why my heart is hurting, but I can explain why this burn hurts. Self-harm became my validation.

Some of my parts engage in self-harm. For my younger parts, a lot of it is trauma re-enacting. For my older parts, most of it is for emotional release, as it is for me. There are a lot of times that I've self-harmed and not remembered doing it. Before I knew what dissociation was and before I was diagnosed, I just assumed it was because I was crazy. I came to learn that my lack of memory was actually because I was dissociated.

Other parts who don't self-harm are scared and don't understand it. It's been really difficult to get a handle on things when all my parts have such different attitudes and understanding. I try to remember that when I am damaging my body, I am also damaging their body.

My self-harm has decreased dramatically since I ran away from home, but it is still something I struggle with daily. The thoughts and urges are still there, and there are times when I do act them out. It scares me, because a lot of times I don't feel fully in control. Sometimes, I am so numb that I can't feel any pain at all, even when the injuries are severe. I fear that someday I may go too far and not realize it until it's too late.

*

ALICIA PETTIS
Alicia was diagnosed with 40
personalities in 2015 at age 16

Between the ages of eight and sixteen I engaged in self-harm. I would burn myself and claim it was an accident, or cut my arm up and claim I fell and scraped it. I would also starve and hit myself. I did those things because it was terrifying not staying in control, and having other people tell me that the people I would talk about, my alters, weren't real. Self-harm made me focus on the pain and stay present. Sometimes my alters would have to step in and stop it because it was getting too dangerous. Other times I was able to get pretty far, or one of my harmful alters would guide me into trying to end things.

Some of my alters used to self-harm as well, as a way to cope with some of the things that were happening in my life, but they have since found alternatives. Others hated it, and hated that I would do it; they tried to constantly reassure me that self-harm wasn't a route I should take, but I never listened to them. Now we all try to function without the thoughts of self-harm. When one of us reverts to self-harm, it's not as serious as it once was. We do get help for those of us who battle with the self-harm urges, though.

*

SUNSHINE PURCELL
Denise was diagnosed with 17
personalities in 1995 at age 30

My self-harm is how I perceive myself. I hate myself, feel disgust, and loathe myself. I can't feel love. I have to ask in order to know. My body shut down that part a long time ago. I don't know how to allow it in. I feel unworthy, unlovable. I don't know what I am here on Earth. I'm not bitter at all, I'm just a shell when it comes to myself. People say you can't love others unless you love yourself. For me, that's not true. I can love others just fine. I can empathize and show I care, be the best friend to a fault. I just don't know how to receive it or how to understand my good points. I am very surprised at compliments and ask why, or point out my flaws. I feel like an alien on this planet, and I'm here for others, to help others, no matter the cost.

*

ERICKA REEVE
Ericka was diagnosed with over 25
personalities in 2013 at age 26

I don't self-harm. I scratched often as a child and I still do, but it isn't because I want to harm myself; I'm trying to calm myself. Some of my parts have self harmed; some struggle with it still, but we're working on this together. I've come to realize that specific parts handle the physical pain—it's one of their purposes. They either share it or individually hold it, depending upon the part. One of their many necessary talents, unfortunately.

*

CHRIS ROBIN
Chris was diagnosed with at least
7 personalities in 2013 at age 49

I am not one to inflict physical harm on myself, like cutting, but I engage in self-harm behaviors such as drinking alcohol, smoking cigarettes, abusing drugs, or isolating and hiding from the world. I've attempted suicide, and I think about it often. I think several parts of me blame themselves for hurting me or wanting to hurt themselves. A few parts are positive and encouraging, but other parts are very negative and hopeless. Finding ways for all of me to come together and use all their strengths is very hard, but I am trying. It's extremely hard to find healthy ways to release emotions.

*

QUINN ROSE
Quinn was diagnosed with 9
personalities in 2016 at age 21

I don't personally self-harm, but one of my alters does. I wake up to marks when in a depressive state. On multiple occasions I have almost died due to being anemic from the blood loss.

*

AYA SAKURA
Aya has been living with 7
personalities since childhood

In my fourth year of high school, when I was sixteen, I had a week-long trip provided by our school as part of the program just before summer vacation. This was also the time when I really started noticing my blackouts and gaps in my memory. I finally connected the voices to my blackouts, and got scared of my voices. I really did not like the idea of the trip, and was really scared of it. At some point there was so much emotional stress built up that one of my alters—Brianna, I think—used the nails to make long scratches on the back of my body. She did this so violently that it started bleeding, and I had wounds on my back. The wounds lasted quite long, even though my body heals quite fast, since she kept opening them after crusts formed. The pain was a way of keeping herself grounded and keeping me away.

My classmates and the teachers who were with me on the trip noticed the wounds. I had foolishly worn a top instead of a shirt. I thought I was sunburned. The thought that I could have wounds on my shoulders didn't even cross my mind, as I trusted myself to never do such a thing. My classmates found them weird, but no one asked questions as far as I can remember. I never heard anything about them from my teachers, but that can also be because one of my alters handled it. My parents found out while we were on vacation, when I again wore a top, this time backless, since I thought everything had healed. My parents were shocked and asked questions, of course. But I brushed them off by telling them I did not know where they came from and claimed it must have been something from the trip, like a rough wall I had been leaning against. It's been a few years now, but I still have faint scars on my back and shoulders. I hope that none of my alters do this again in order to relieve emotions or stress.

I do not currently engage in self-harm as an emotional release. I used to swim twice a week for about fourteen years, and would be in great trouble if someone saw scars or wounds, since I also taught elementary-aged children in the pool. So I (and my alters) learned to suppress the urges but because of that, my alters have now developed equally harmful behavior. I am not comfortable with having wounds or being in pain, so I am really scared of harming myself, which is why I'm not engaging in self-harm.

I have two active alters nowadays, and both of them are harming the body in another way. Brianna is a model in the inner world and does not eat. If she feels like fainting and really needs to eat, she eats fruit or drinks smoothies. Sometimes she can be convinced to eat something else by her husband, Clive. She does drink water, caffeinated coffee, and alcohol—lots of alcohol. Brianna told me that this is done to relax and to stop herself from thinking. Clive smokes in both the inner and outer world. He is cutting down on cigarettes currently, and I'm very proud of him for that. I don't know why he smokes, but I guess it's a way to relax and relieve stress for him, since he doesn't drink alcohol. He gets really sick and stays away when alcohol is involved.

As for myself, I try to be healthy and as normal as possible by not smoking, drinking only a little, and not hurting myself in a way that would have a longer-lasting effect. I do push my nails into my arms or hands when I am really stressed out or when I need to stay as grounded as possible, but I take great care by always making sure my nails never break my skin. Most of the time the marks fade away in a few hours.

I really do not like that Clive smokes as I dislike cigarettes from the bottom of my heart, nor do I like that Brianna uses alcohol to relieve stress and emotion, since alcohol can be dangerous in the large quantities she drinks. Right now I'm trying to work together with them to get them to use healthy coping skills and mechanisms.

*

FLOSS SCOTT
Floss was diagnosed with at least
4 personalities in 2016 at age 48

I've never tried to self-harm by cutting myself, as I'm too afraid of any form of sharp implements near or on my skin. I tend to punish myself rather than cut, as it's less painful physically. I self-harm by feeding myself negative thoughts. For example, if I've been rejected, it really hurts me so I'll look for a reason as to why. I'll mentally tell myself I'm worthless, and that's why I've been rejected. So in order to justify the rejection, I punish myself by justifying why I was rejected. I hope this makes sense.

*

KERRYJANE VOTH
Kerryjane was diagnosed with
35 alters in 2013 at age 53

We don't engage in self-harm. We don't turn to drinking, smoking or drugs. We do turn to food at times, mostly chocolate though in moderation. But what we do is turn to our service dog, our therapist, and friends, in that order. We use physical activities like lots of walks, hikes and bike riding, play or study, write music, and mindfulness meditation. When we really need a good dose of relief, we spend time at a friend's home on the lake. After several days of peace and quiet, walking the beach, and playing in the surf, along with my friend's loving kindness, we feel renewed.

*

CHAPTER FOURTEEN

The Face in the Mirror

Life is a mirror and will reflect back to the thinker
what he thinks into it. -ERNEST HOLMES

DID is often portrayed in the movies as alters wearing dramatically different styles. Because some alters are male and some are female, and some are non-gender, picking out clothes and deciding on which fingernail polish or hairstyle can certainly be a challenge, but not always. Who decides what to wear each day? Who do you see when you look in the mirror?

*

ADRIANNE ALLEN-LANG
Adrianne was diagnosed with 10
personalities in 2015 at age 18

We all see the host. When someone is out, small things change automatically, but sometimes they'll go change or put on a wig.

*

GAIL BUSWELL
Gail was diagnosed with 13
personalities in 2002 at age 24

We have always needed to conform to uniformity, so dressing was never an issue. We all like to wear our hair differently, and just one of us likes to wear makeup. We don't own a mirror, and try to avoid seeing the body. We all have very different self-images and seeing the body only causes confusion and upset.

*

KATT HART
Katt was diagnosed with hundreds
of personalities in 2011 at age 20

Figuring out clothes is an absolute pain. There's usually some debate every time we get dressed over what to wear, or there's some other issue like gender or the body looking wrong, or our weight that bothers some of us. We have a lot of different clothes, so most alters have things they're at least slightly more comfortable wearing. The main issues come when there are multiple alters around at the same time who have different styles. We usually go for jeans and a T-shirt, but some of the others want to wear a dress or a skirt. Some like revealing clothing and crop tops, but those who have trouble with our weight or the body's gender get upset about it. Most of our alters are male or nonbinary, so the body being considered female is a big issue for us. We used to have a chest binder, but our chronic pain made that very hard to comfortably wear for more than an hour or two. Instead, we now have a lot of baggy T-shirts and hoodies that help hide the body's figure. The baggy clothes also come in handy for the people with weight problems, but they don't want clothes that are too baggy in case that makes us look fatter in their eyes.

The alters see themselves in the mirror unless they purposely look at the body, which they often have to do while getting ready to make sure the body is presentable to the outside world, rather than what we think we look like. Makeup, unfortunately, has to be done every time we leave the house or have someone coming over, because of insecurities of some alters. If we don't have makeup on, they'll have panic attacks and refuse to go anywhere or see anyone.

Our hair is an interesting dilemma. Since it's quite short, it's usually styled vaguely the same way when we go out. But the color changes all the time, and we can't seem to decide on one color to have for long. We also can't get haircuts very easily. Last time we did, one of the boys got our hair cut short and upset half of the others, who wanted it longer. There's always an ongoing debate on how to have our hair, but whoever ends up at the hairdresser is often the one to decide, and that causes a lot of upset and arguments almost every time.

*

AMELIA JOUBERT
Amelia was diagnosed with 12
personalities in 2013 at age 15

Hello! I am Scarlet and I am going to answer this question, since I'm kind of the fashionista of our system. Despite how some media portray it, we don't change into a completely new outfit every time we switch. Our general rule is that whoever is out when it's time to get dressed and ready for the day gets to pick what we wear for the day.

I'll give you a little rundown of how some of us like to dress. I love girly clothes like dresses and fancy blouses. Amelia says I dress like a prep, but I love it! May and Amelia are into the alternative look and both like to wear band tees and colored jeggings. Jax usually wears tank tops from the mens' section of the store, and a pair of basketball shorts. Ahina likes to wear Southern clothes like boots and checkered shirts.

When it comes to hair, Amelia, Ahina, and I like it down. May usually puts it in a ponytail, and Jax usually wears it up in a beanie. Sometimes John will come out and braid it, too. Jax doesn't wear makeup and Amelia rarely does. I love makeup and it's a coping skill for me, so even if Amelia gets dressed in the morning, I often come out to do the makeup.

*

AMANDA LINEBACK
Amanda was diagnosed with hundreds
of personalities in 2013 at age 31

We have always just dressed for the role we had to take on each day. We aren't consistently out for enough time to come up with a clothing schedule. Whoever is out gets to pick what the body wears, and we all agree. When we put on makeup, the little girls sometimes try to take over, and that never goes very well. If a teenager spent two hours getting dolled up and a three-year-old takes over during the finishing touches, it causes a huge fight.

*

JANE MACDONALD
Jane was diagnosed with 3 personalities in
2014 at age 35, and currently has 6 alters

How I dress or do my hair and makeup has never been a problem. I do not have much communication with my alters, so if they were concerned or unhappy with my appearance I'm not sure that I would know unless they changed it, which they have not. Occasionally I find things in my wardrobe that one of the alters has purchased, and it may not be my style, so I simply choose not to wear it. Of course it makes it easy for me that all my alters are female, so there is no difficulty in terms of gender roles. I am honestly grateful that these things are not an issue for me, as I seem to have enough struggles to deal with.

*

CRYSTALIE MATULEWICZ
Crystalie was diagnosed with dissociative
identity disorder in 2015 at age 29

I have to wear a uniform for work, so for four or five days out of each week I don't have to worry about disagreements about what we wear, because we really don't have a choice. I actually like it that way, as it saves a lot of time in the mornings because we don't have to switch out different clothes.

My parts and I have different styles and like different colors, which can cause conflict when I'm not in uniform. Aside from work days, rarely do I have a day when the first outfit I put on is the one I end up leaving the house with. I only own two pairs of jeans, so that keeps any changes to a minimum. But shirts—I own such an array of shirts. Dressy shirts, flowery shirts, tank tops, costume hoodies, and dozens of T-shirts. I even have a hoodie that turns into Spiderman. I change my shirt at least three times before leaving the house, and sometimes as many as seven or eight times. I pick something out to wear, put it on, and am pulled to put on something completely different. Sometimes I end up in something I would never wear, but wear it because another part wants to.

My style is relatively simple. I have a fascination with Superman. He gave me hope as a child that I would escape one day, so I have a lot of Superman T-shirts that I like to wear. Really, I would wear a Superman T-shirt every day if I could. But my parts don't necessarily share the same likes, so we end up wearing different things.

My parts and I have different favorite colors, which affects what we choose to wear. I like black and different shades of blue, and don't stray away from that much at all. One of my parts likes green; not regular or dark green, but shockingly bright lime green. Another part likes pink. This is particularly troublesome for me, because I detest the color pink. It annoyed me one day when I looked in my closet to find I had acquired a pink polka dot backpack and a pink shirt. It was difficult for me to keep them, but I realized that my parts have different likes, and that I have to allow them to be themselves, even if it doesn't always match up with who I am. I do have male parts, so there are times when we dress that lean toward an androgynous style. The T-shirts help a lot with that. I don't use purses or handbags, but have a collection of backpacks in various colors, so we can stay more gender ambiguous.

Footwear isn't much of an issue, but not by choice. I wear a men's size eleven, so footwear selection is quite limited to what's available in men's sizes. Sometimes I get white sneakers and let parts color on them. It's fun for them to do, while also letting them show their style, which is otherwise limited because of our size.

I don't wear makeup, and don't own much aside from the essentials for the rare special occasion, so that has never been a source of disagreement between my parts and me. Hair is another story. I have naturally wavy hair. I prefer to wear it straightened, and I use a lot of conditioner to keep my hair weighed down. Other parts like our hair curly (I had naturally curly hair when I was younger). It is difficult for me, because seeing my hair that way brings up unpleasant childhood memories that I have yet to work through. It's hard to explain to a younger part, who is essentially a child, why we can't wear our hair that way. They don't understand it like I do, because they don't have the same associations that I do.

We've had an array of hair colors over the years, everything from blonde to black to pink. I'm open to allowing different colors that other parts may want, and fortunately my workplaces have had lax rules when it comes to that. We've also had really long hair and short hair. I have a part who comes out when I'm angry and has a tendency to chop off our hair. It's helpful in a way, because I never have to go to a salon to get my hair done, though sometimes I end up with much shorter hair than I prefer. I have to work with it even though it doesn't fit my style. I've had to learn to let little things go. Whatever I wear, whatever my hair color or length, that doesn't affect who we are.

*

ALICIA PETTIS
Alicia was diagnosed with 40
personalities in 2015 at age 16

Dressing in the morning is interesting. Most of the time it's me who gets dressed, but if not, then I can tell who was out by the way I look. Loose, baggy clothing, combat boots, and no makeup is most likely Sophia. She dresses like that in case she needs to get into a fight. Dark makeup, dark clothing, and my bangs showing is Larissa. She has a gothic style that definitely shows itself when she's out. When it comes to male alters, they try to dress the way they feel comfortable. Whether that's in a flannel shirt and some jeans or in a full suit—it's up to them, and to my wardrobe.

All of my alters see me when they look into a mirror, at least that's what I've been told. They know they won't look fully like themselves to the outside world, and that kind of upsets them. That's why I allow my alters to dress the way they like. Also, if my hair has any type of ribbon or hairclip, that's most likely Kayleigh. It honestly can be any one of my littles, but the feeling would be more Kay than anyone else.

*

SUNSHINE PURCELL
Denise was diagnosed with 17
personalities in 1995 at age 30

Me, the main host, usually sets the dress of the day depending on what needs to be done, or if we have to leave the house. Knowing that not all of them are girls, I will wear flannels or sweatpants or nongender attire like baseball hats, etc. When I do my makeup, it's habit. I only put it in for public appearances unless the women are feeling extra feminine. I don't look in the mirror; none of us really do. I know that the little one, Sarah, says sometimes it confuses them, because they know how they look. They all share the body, but they all have a distinct look; for some, it shows in their eyes and, of course, mannerisms and voices.

*

ERICKA REEVE
Ericka was diagnosed with over 25
personalities in 2013 at age 26

Well, this depends on who's around, I suppose. It does vary, as everything else seems to. I dress very differently from some of them, and they do from each other as well. Jynx regularly does my hair and makeup because she worked in the entertainment and fashion industry. No, she wasn't a stripper. That's not what we meant by entertainment industry.

If we're co-conscious, she respects that I rarely go full glam. But she is quite talented. I'm a T-shirt and jeans kind of person but she helps me dress up that look in a more adult way, even though she's ten years my junior. When Jynx looks in the mirror she sees herself unless she is doing makeup on me or one of the others. Some of the younger parts or littles adore her, so she does something fun or special for them from time to time. A very creative pre-teen part was upset the other day (I say the other day when I've no real certainty of the time). Anyway, she was upset and Jynx turned her into a cartoon puppy, complete with ears painted using a few of her cream eye shadows. She wasn't pleased about doing it, but this little needed help, and Jynx knew she could calm her by doing this.

Different styles among all of us, including the different genders, are very tricky at times. I'm only just now learning of a male teen part, and he came to be seen in a spectacularly destructive manner. I'm told he was shouting at our mother part, Minny, that he is NOT a girl and to stop dressing him that way. I'm learning how to handle all these things, and juggling is something we excel at, but not me, so we work together to ensure that everyone is okay.

*

CHRIS ROBIN
Chris was diagnosed with at least
7 personalities in 2013 at age 49

Honestly, I have never thought about this question. I pretty much have had my hair this way for thirty years, and I don't wear makeup, so that doesn't seem to be a problem. I've had moments in my life when I have shaved my head, colored my hair or etched shapes into my hair, but those thoughts come and go. I've never really cared much about my appearance or how I dress. I dress for comfort and for what I'm doing, not to impress anyone, including my parts. I have been approached by my bosses and told that, in the capacity of the job, I do I need to look more formal. It is very difficult to shop for clothes, because I really don't know my style or what I want to look like. It might be because all the parts of me have different tastes. The same is true for choosing a place to eat.

Looking in a mirror is a different subject. I rarely purposely make eye contact with myself. When I do, sometimes I don't know who is looking back at me. Sometimes the person in the mirror is a stranger, and the person I had been earlier that day is invisible to me. I don't ever really see myself the way others see me. I don't like looking at myself, probably because I don't know who I really am.

*

QUINN ROSE
Quinn was diagnosed with 9
personalities in 2016 at age 21

Each one has a different style and will try to dress accordingly. Sometimes it's subtle, depending on whether we have to see family. Danielle will dress baggy and guyish, Raven in pinup, and Carley wears long skirts and sweaters. Trixie wears anything that's fun, and Luna in barely anything at all. Yuno wears cutesy clothing. Roxy wears a leather jacket and bra and pants. Stuff like that.

*

AYA SAKURA
Aya has been living with 7
personalities since childhood

Most of the time I just wake up, dress myself and do my hair and makeup according to how much time I have and how much effort I want to put into it. I mostly end up with a bit of makeup and the clothing I feel best in that day. I tend to stay a bit neutral, something like a pair of jeans, a shirt and a blouse.

For days when either Brianna or Clive wake up, they mostly choose, just like me, the clothing they feel best in. They also both do their hair differently. For Brianna it's mostly skirts, heels, jewelry, accessories, and a full face of makeup. She likes to show off that she's a woman and is proud of that. She is a model and singer in the inner world, and really cares about appearances because of that.

Clive tends to go for a jeans and a sweater combination without any makeup at all, since he doesn't really care much about his appearance. He sometimes experiences gender dysphoria and then tries to hide the fact that he is in a female body. When he's got a choice, he'll change into jeans if he's wearing a skirt. This helps me a lot, because I can almost see by clothing and makeup who was out in the morning. If I know that, I can also, for example, figure out if I have eaten, whether I need to buy food for lunch, and where I might have been and what I was doing the past few hours.

I don't always feel comfortable with the way Brianna dresses and the fact that Clive doesn't wear any makeup. Most of the time when I come out after either one has dressed up, I go to the bathroom to either take off all the jewelry and accessories, or to put on a bit of makeup. The latter only happens when I've been lucky enough that Clive took makeup with him or if it just stayed in my bag from another day. When I am feeling really uncomfortable, even after trying to make myself feel comfortable, I just try to hide in the back of the classroom until eventually one of them takes over.

On days when I feel very fuzzy, when I don't know for sure who I am, or if my alters want to dress like me for some reason, I have a complete set of clothing in my closet. This is a set I would normally pick myself, so that my alters don't have to mess up my closet trying to find out what I would normally wear.

*
FLOSS SCOTT
Floss was diagnosed with at least
4 personalities in 2016 at age 48

When each of my alters appears, they normally will just see that alter looking in the mirror. I have these styles: Sophisticated. Sexy. Boyish. Don't care. Each style will appear depending on which person is leading that morning. I have changed alters during the day and wondered why on earth I'm dressed like this, and will go change clothes. My makeup will normally stay the same; I guess they all like it. All my alters are female, but I think that there might have been a boy when I was younger.

*

KERRYJANE VOTH
Kerryjane was diagnosed with
35 alters in 2013 at age 53

This is a touchy subject for some of my alters, because I have both male and female alters consisting of both children and a few adults. None of them are very comfortable dressing in the others' clothes. So trying to find something to wear each day, something that everyone will at least agree they can tolerate, can become difficult. The worst that can happen is that one alter gets to dress the way he or she likes, and once out of the house when it's too late to change, another alter takes over and doesn't feel like the clothes are appropriate or comfortable. This happened once when we were at a dance in Toronto. We let one of our females shop for the clothes to wear to the dance. She had a great time picking out just the right dress and the system seemed fine with the choice until the night of the dance. A male alter came online and was fit to be tied when he found himself in a dress at a dance and in public. He was horrified and terribly uncomfortable. Since then, we haven't been able to leave the house in a dress for fear that one of our males would find himself inappropriately dressed in public.

It's been a compromise with clothes, not too girly and not too masculine. As a system, we've been trying to walk a middle road. But we still feel the pull from some alters who would very much love to dress either really feminine or really masculine. The alters look forward to the day when they can just dress whatever way they want and it will be no big deal.

We don't wear much makeup anymore. It seems to be easier on the skin. We all agreed that getting dreadlocks would work for everyone, because some like the length, while others like not having to fuss with hairdryers and curling irons anymore. It's also unisex, depending on how you style them.

*

CHAPTER FIFTEEN

Confessing our Fears

The oldest and strongest emotion of mankind is fear,
and the oldest and strongest kind of fear is fear of
the unknown. -H. P. LOVECRAFT

Fear is a natural emotion, but those who live with dissociative identity disorder can have magnified fears, especially when coupled with post-traumatic stress disorder. Different alters and parts can fear different things, including fear of oneself and the outside world, fear of the past and the future. For those with PTSD, flashbacks and other post-traumatic symptoms can magnify fear even further. What part of living with dissociative identity disorder do you fear the most?

*

ADRIANNE ALLEN-LANG
Adrianne was diagnosed with 10
personalities in 2015 at age 18

I fear that I'm not going to find a life partner who can handle it, to be honest. I can't handle it most days, so I know I'm asking a lot of another; but one day we'll find someone who loves us all.

*

GAIL BUSWELL
Gail was diagnosed with 13
personalities in 2002 at age 24

I fear always living in this hell. I am scared that my body will not survive the memories of the related trauma. Not suicide; that the body will just say that enough is enough, I can't cope with the body memories, the flashbacks and the rapid switching among alters. Every day we join the dots a little more, and it is so painful. I fear being deemed crazy, stupid, weak, incapable, disabled, too much, not enough. If fear people I love walking away or being taken from me. I fear never finding someone who will stay. I fear never being able to hold down a job again because I cannot remember what I learned yesterday. I fear suddenly not knowing what is going on and wanting my mum.

*

KATT HART
Katt was diagnosed with hundreds
of personalities in 2011 at age 20

Most of us think the hardest and scariest part of having DID is the abuse and trauma connected to it. Most of us are so terrified of the day when we finally learn the truth of it all. How will we cope with that, and what do we do with that sort of information? It's terrifying. Knowing that our brain separated all of this off for a reason, but we have to remember at least some of it to be able to heal and move forward, is absolutely terrifying.

The time loss and disconnect from our body and the world is scary, but those are things we can deal with, or have methods to prevent them or stop it from being as bad. The trauma is something we can't just stop from happening any more. It isn't something we can find ways to prevent; it's something we have to live and work with, and integrate into who we are in order to continue living.

If we had a therapist, that would be a different matter; we'd have a professional to help us cope with this in healthy ways, a professional who could monitor how much we're learning and how to manage it. But we don't, and we're unsure when or if we will.

*

AMELIA JOUBERT
Amelia was diagnosed with 12
personalities in 2013 at age 15

Scarlet answering. For me the hardest part of DID is having to share a body and a life with other people. Amelia and I are out the most, and we both want to have a dream wedding, kids, etc. Amelia is into girls and I am into guys, so it's not like we could share someone. I don't know if I would even want to do that. This is something I think about a lot. I mean, sure, we all have our own body in the inner world, but my true love is not in there, and I don't know if I will get a chance to find him out here. It's either me or Amelia; that's how it seems. I want kids who will know me for myself, and call me mommy—just me. So for me, that is the hardest part. But on the flip side I love my inner family and I don't know what I would do without them.

*

AMANDA LINEBACK
Amanda was diagnosed with hundreds
of personalities in 2013 at age 31

Living with dissociative identity disorder is not frightening to me. The person *we* have become, the person *we* have always been, the person whom people have known, did not change because of a diagnosis. I have always lived with DID, I just didn't know that I was a multiple. To me, what is scary about having DID is the horrific amounts of torture I was forced to endure as a small child. It is terrifying to think about being so abused that your brain has to take you away and create someone else in order to endure the abuse. It's abuse so awful, that it's like being tortured to death, except you didn't die physically. The person I was born as was taken away. It didn't physically kill me, but it did take something from me that I can never get back.

It's horrible knowing that everyone inside me was created during trauma, as a response to trauma, to avoid triggers, or to avoid being affected by triggers. There are parts of me who have only known torture and pain. There are parts who have never felt happiness. It's scary knowing that people who were supposed to protect me abused me instead, and made me feel like I had done something to deserve it, or believe I was born inherently unlovable.

The way I'm treated by most doctors, nurses, law enforcement, and even most mental health facilities is frightening. I'm ridiculed, mocked, interrogated, and often accused of being on drugs when I go to the hospital for help. I went to the hospital once for having seizures after a concussion, and a doctor abruptly stopped my CT scan to say that my symptoms were from the drugs in my system. So the medicine prescribed for me by one doctor is used against me by another.

Having to be my own advocate and handle stressful situations is a nightmare. What I actually want to say never comes out appropriate enough, and sometimes the people who are supposed to help me just walk out. I feel as if my cycle of abuse is on an eternal loop of being abused and then traumatized by doctors because of my abuse. The overall lack of compassion I've faced over the last four years disgusts me. It is disheartening to realize how mean and insensitive people are toward one another, and how self-involved, hypocritical, and manipulative they can be.

I've always known that I am a loving, caring, empathetic and funny individual. It hurts to be treated differently after being diagnosed, and realize how easily the people you're closest to will turn their backs and act like they don't know you. I've been manipulated so much that I start to question myself. Having DID itself is not scary. The way I am treated by people when they find out my diagnosis, however, is what frightens me.

*

JANE MACDONALD
Jane was diagnosed with 3 personalities in
2014 at age 35, and currently has 6 alters

I think the thing I fear the most about having DID is the uncertainty that it brings. Life, in general, is full of uncertainties, but when you have other personalities, this takes on a whole new meaning. For one thing, I never know who is going to come out, what they are going to say, or what they are going to do. I don't have much awareness of my other personalities and have no control over when they come out or what happens when they are out. I have come to, for instance, standing in the middle of a road with cars honking at me to move. I had no idea how long I had been there. I worry that if something like this happens again, I could be seriously injured. As another example, I have one alter who self-harms quite severely. I am always afraid of how badly she will harm me, and what she may say to someone else. I know she intensely dislikes my psychiatrist and tried to convince another alter to attack him (thankfully, unsuccessfully). I worry about how she will react if she comes out in one of our sessions. Will she say or do something to hurt my psychiatrist? If she does, will he dump me as a client and tell me he cannot work with me? I wouldn't blame him. I have heard of other psychiatrists or therapists who dumped their DID clients for a lot less than that.

Since I'm largely unaware of what happens when my alters are out, I'm left trying to figure out what happened during the day. Did they do or say anything inappropriate that I have to answer for? Did they hurt someone, say something mean, or commit to something like a meeting or a job that I don't want to do? Did they spend a lot of money on items I can't afford? It's an uneasy feeling to realize that you've lost time and have no clue what happened for the last few hours, or even days. It's like trying to piece together a puzzle without even knowing where to find the pieces.

There is also uncertainty as to how others will react if one of my other personalities comes out in public. Will people assume it is just me having an off day? Will they suspect I have DID? Will they think I am schizophrenic? Will they be accepting and respectful? Will they ignore me? Will they be critical or confused? What questions will they ask me about what happened, and how do I answer them? Although a few of the people I've told have been very supportive and accepting, not everyone is like that. Some accuse you of faking it for the attention. Others are confused and don't know what to think. I'm afraid not only of the questions they ask, but also the questions they don't. It is the unsaid things that perhaps frighten me the most.

*

CRYSTALIE MATULEWICZ
Crystalie was diagnosed with dissociative
identity disorder in 2015 at age 29

I fear the memories. It's taken me so much time to process just a fraction of what I went through. I worry about what trauma my parts are still hiding from me. Do I want to know? Can I handle knowing? I sometimes worry that the memories will be too much for me to handle, and I'll shut down completely.

I fear for our future. I worry about getting fired from my job or being kicked out of school because of DID. I worry about whether I'll ever be able to work full time. I fear not being able to support myself financially. I am barely scraping by, and fear being homeless because I had to leave my family to keep myself and my parts safe from harm.

I fear getting lost inside and never finding my way out. I fear dissociating so badly that I can never come back. I fear losing so much time that I can no longer function. I fear getting so wrapped up in all of my parts that I will never find my own identity.

I fear failing at therapy. I fear that my therapist will give up, that she will realize that I am too broken to fix. I fear that maybe I really am just crazy. Maybe there is no help for me, for us.

I fear death. Over seventy percent of people with DID attempt suicide. I've made multiple attempts and, by some miracle, have survived—though not unscathed. I spend my days anxiously waiting for when those feelings will come back; they always do. I fear that I will try again and not make it out alive. I fear that one of my parts will succeed at taking our life, because they don't realize that killing themselves means killing us all.

I fear society. I worry what people will think of me when they find out I have DID. Will they call me crazy? Will they run away from me? Will they accuse me of things I've never done? Will they see me for what I am—a human being—or will they think I'm a monster?

When the sky is covered in dark clouds, people forget that the sun exists behind them; they only focus on the darkness. I fear that no matter what good I do, my diagnosis will be like those dark clouds. I have the potential to accomplish so many great things, but I fear my diagnosis will discredit any work I do. In many ways, it already has. I had to give up my dream because the community that is supposed to be the most understanding is the least accepting of people like us.

I fear myself.
I fear the world.
I live in fear.
My parts live in fear.
It's a fear that never goes away.

*

ALICIA PETTIS
Alicia was diagnosed with 40
personalities in 2015 at age 16

Growing up, I always thought it was normal to lose time or have other people frequently mistake your name. What scared me the most is the fact that that wasn't the case. No normal person went through such things. I also find schoolwork hard because of my alters misplacing work, or me missing tons of information because they're stubborn and won't show me what I missed while I was out.

I do enjoy some aspects related to having DID, such as going inside the system when I need to do chores. They've never been my favorite thing to do, and they're also a slight trigger to me. Another example would be losing time with my homework, and when I come back it's all done for me. I don't enjoy losing time when it's important to me, but at the same time I understand that it means something isn't right and I need a break. Most of the time, however, they come out just to have fun and be themselves.

*

SUNSHINE PURCELL
Denise was diagnosed with 17
personalities in 1995 at age 30

I fear that people will still not understand why this happens. We need to develop a therapeutic way to help with symptoms. We need to listen to the individual—not disregard what they say or how they feel because it doesn't fall within the usual standards. DID is real and more common than we want to admit. It's masked by misdiagnoses, and people don't know what to do.

*

ERICKA REEVE
Ericka was diagnosed with over
25 personalities in 2013 at age 26

I fear missing more of my life or just being gone completely some day. If something awful were to occur now, I imagine I would be gone again for a very long time—a year maybe, or longer. I fear them just completely taking my life one day. Some of the biggest obstacles is that we've spent my entire life hiding. Now we are working toward being more open with friends and people we care about. That's a short-ish list, but it's causing some crippling anxiety as of late.

Now that I know I have DID, some things are amusing to me and no longer frightening. Pre-diagnosis, it would freak me out when I had no memory of creating various paintings or projects. As an example, I would have no idea where certain new clothes came from, or why I was in a new apartment. That being said, my parts tend to *always* have a reason for the things they do, most of them, at least. The big one for me is that they've kept me (us) alive all these years, but now I want to be able to help them and live harmoniously, and maybe one day openly.

*

CHRIS ROBIN
Chris was diagnosed with at least
7 personalities in 2013 at age 49

Right now I am in fear of everything that has to do with DID, because it is still new to me. I think the thing I fear the most is the possibility that a part of me might take over and I won't be able to know or understand what he or she did, and whether he or she did something bad or illegal. Those lost times are the scariest for me. There are times when I am so far removed from one of my parts that I can feel the real me fading away, and I don't know if I will always be able to get back to my present. The other thing that scares me is how easy it is for my brain to switch and become someone else, and I won't be able to learn to know the difference. However, acknowledging the parts of me and communicating is taking some of that fear away.

*

QUINN ROSE
Quinn was diagnosed with 9
personalities in 2016 at age 21

People don't believe DID exists; they believe I'm just using it as an excuse. They think that my alters will screw up the life I am trying to establish for myself. I fear not knowing if tomorrow I will wake up in a place I don't even know. I fear that I don't truly know everything I have done in my life. I fear I will never get those lost days back. I fear not having control of my own body or mind, and living in darkness most of the time. I fear that people think I can just conveniently alter my memories.

*

AYA SAKURA
Aya has been living with 7
personalities since childhood

The part of living with DID that scares me most is regaining my consciousness after an alter has been out and seeing what has happened. Blackouts are great in the sense that I do not have to be around and it feels like I am sleeping. But I have no sense of time passing, just like when one is sleeping. I am very scared of my blackouts, because I don't have any idea what happened, and I don't know how much time has passed or what I am doing. I could be gone for years, and I would be scared that I had missed so much that I would not be able to pick up my life anymore.

I'm also very scared that my alters hurt people I care about. I really care very much about the people who are closest to me, and I couldn't forgive my alters if they did or said something cruel to my friends or family. Even though Makah made important decisions for a long time, I'm scared of my alters making important decisions and changing the course of my life. This brings me to something else which I fear very much. I really fear not being able to pick up my life again after I have been away for a while because I've been gone too long or my alters did something.

My other big fear is not being able to come back. Every time I come back I think, my god, thank heavens I was able to come back. I see not coming back as dying, in a way. I'm not really afraid of dying, but the scary thing is that I won't really be dead and I'll be trapped in a struggle to come back.

*

FLOSS SCOTT
Floss was diagnosed with at least
4 personalities in 2016 at age 48

With my knowledge of DID, I fear doing some of the things I've done in the past, and fear the dangers I may have put myself in. I also fear being rejected by others. As soon as I told my husband that I had DID, he read up about it and then left me. That was the worst feeling ever, and I don't know how I'm going to overcome that. Now I fear that if I meet someone, they'll do the same, too. This is definitely my worst fear, but it's not the end of the world.

*

KERRYJANE VOTH
Kerryjane was diagnosed with
35 alters in 2013 at age 53

What I fear the most about living with DID is old age and dying. I worry that I will be left in a bed somewhere, and no one will understand that there is so much more going on inside me. I worry that when the time comes for this body to pass away, not all of our alters will understand or even know what is going on, and will be afraid, and there will be no one there to comfort them if there is no longer co-consciousness.

I worry that as I get older that I may be compromised through illness and be misdiagnosed with dementia or worse. I don't want to be pumped full of drugs, because not all of our alters react well nor need the drug and have an adverse reaction (which has happened in the past). I'm also fearful of living, because I'm not able to work and try to survive on a meager pension. I worry about whether I will have enough food to eat, or enough gas in the car to get to therapy. I don't have disposable income, so making plans to join friends for activities can be embarrassing or unattainable, leaving me at home most of the time.

There is a very deep loneliness that comes with DID, because of the difficulty with attachment and our cultural stigma toward those with mental health issues.

*

CHAPTER SIXTEEN

Managing a Family

Each day of our lives we make deposits in the
memory banks of our children. -CHARLES R.
SWINDOLL

Some individuals living with dissociative identity disorder have partners, spouses, and even a family. If you have children, how has raising them been impacted by your diagnosis?

*

ADRIANNE ALLEN-LANG
Adrianne was diagnosed with 10
personalities in 2015 at age 18

My son isn't old enough yet to understand.

*

KATT HART
Katt was diagnosed with hundreds
of personalities in 2011 at age 20

We have no children, and we're quite scared of the day when we may have children. If we did, then I think we would probably be open about our DID from an early age but leave out the upsetting details until they were old enough to understand. Most alters get along with our partner though. We're very lucky to be in a relationship with another person who has DID, so our alters interact, help, and understand one another. Of course there are clashes sometimes, and we try to keep alters away from each other who don't get along. But for the most part it works better than any other relationship we've been in, because this is the first time we've been with someone else who genuinely understands.

*

AMELIA JOUBERT
Amelia was diagnosed with 12
personalities in 2013 at age 15

Scarlet answering. I don't have kids, but I really want them. I know Amelia does too. I wish there was a way Amelia and I could each have our own family, but I don't see that happening. The main twelve of us get along with our friends and family pretty well. Our little K loves our mom, and they talk a lot. May doesn't like adults who are not in our system, so she usually doesn't come out around them. Both Amelia and I are close with friends and family, and the others are on a friendly first-name basis. Most of us, however, are very close with our friends, Kayla and Jacob.

*

AMANDA LINEBACK
Amanda was diagnosed with hundreds
of personalities in 2013 at age 31

I made the decision to have the children stay with their dad for a year when I was first diagnosed. I missed them badly but knew that being a good mom meant that I needed to do what was the best for them, and I could barely piece together what happened each day. Their dad had them through the week and my mom would keep them on the weekends. I spent the night with them on the weekends, so we all had a babysitter.

Having to admit that I wasn't stable enough to take care of my babies was the hardest thing I have ever done. I think that more than anything, the way I felt about myself as a mother was weakened when I first got my diagnosis. It was a blow to my self-image, and it was very hard to not get even more depressed thinking that I could possibly be a letdown to my children. I wanted everything to be perfect for them, and it hurt knowing that my children were going to be exposed to the residual effects of my childhood abuse.

The way I raise my children and the things I teach them and talk to them about is because I have dissociative identity disorder. I am honest with my children about everything. In order for them to feel safe, they have to be able to fully trust me. I explain to them how and why I am feeling my emotions, so that they never feel like they are the cause of those emotions. I let them know that it is okay to feel all their emotions, and that all emotions serve a purpose. I have the two most empathetic, compassionate, funny, respectful, and kind children I have ever met. I love you, Jaylin and Jaden.

*

JANE MACDONALD
Jane was diagnosed with 3 personalities in
2014 at age 35, and currently has 6 alters

I do not have any children. Honestly, I am thankful that I do not have children or a romantic partner in my life, because I have a hard enough time understanding and managing my DID on my own, without trying to explain it to others.

*

CRYSTALIE MATULEWICZ
Crystalie was diagnosed with dissociative
identity disorder in 2015 at age 29

I made the decision to not have children while I was in my mid-twenties. That decision was made in part due to health conditions, and in part due to the trauma I had experienced. I expend a tremendous amount of energy just making it through each day. I don't have much energy, either physical or emotional, left to devote to the needs of a family.

Because my mother was my main abuser, I have a lot of trauma reactions connected to mother-child relationships. There is a part of me that fears that I am just like my mother, and that I will hurt a child just like my mother hurt me. I can't even hold a baby or be near someone else's child without being stricken with fear and panic that I am going to hurt the child. The thought of having my own children is terrifying, and something I have decided I cannot go through.

I haven't been involved in any serious relationships. I have difficulty trusting most people. Some of my parts also have trouble trusting others because of what we went through. We have managed to develop a trust with our therapist, but still have difficulty with relationships outside of therapy. We were also taught in childhood not to trust anyone on the outside, and a lot of parts have internalized this belief, which makes it hard for me to get close to anyone.

One part, in particular, does not trust men. He acts out whenever a man gets close to me. It's very confusing for someone when I am talking to them one minute, and hitting them the next for no reason at all. Instead of trying to explain myself, I find it easier to keep my distance from people. Unfortunately, this keeps me isolated. While I do have my parts and I'm not technically alone, I wish I were able to get closer to people on the outside without causing disarray on the inside. I long for a connection that I have not yet been able to find.

*

ALICIA PETTIS
Alicia was diagnosed with 40
personalities in 2015 at age 16

I don't have children, but my alters all enjoy my significant other. He loves them just as much. He claims to see them as family so they don't feel left out if they're outside. All the littles call him Uncle, including Sophia's children who are sixteen. They're twins, and they call him Uncle for reason that cannot be mentioned due to his not wanting it to be out there. My alters also get along with my friends, and see them as their best friend or close acquaintances. If the littles are out and they become scared or frightened of the situation, my significant other or my friends will make sure they have something that makes them feel safe and talk them down from their scared state of mind. If one of the older alters is having a stressful day, they will talk to that alter and see what's going on. It helps the system a lot and takes stress away very easily.

*

SUNSHINE PURCELL
Denise was diagnosed with 17
personalities in 1995 at age 30

All my alters get along with my children. There are a few who don't prefer to deal with kids, so they don't, and that's fine because there are enough who do. What's confusing is that some of my children have a different mother, an alter for that time. It's not really brought up, and I'm not the actual person who mothers them, but I am known as the one who is mostly out so they just call me Mom. But they can tell if Mom isn't out and will say, "Can I talk to Mom for a minute?" As for my significant other, that depends on how we are accepted. There have been sexual gender preferences brought up in the past, but it has to be okay with all the alters or it doesn't work.

*

ERICKA REEVE
Ericka was diagnosed with over 25
personalities in 2013 at age 26

I can't have children, so it hasn't impacted me. We would love to foster children, especially in the LGBT community and those with a societal standard of a difficult background. We have worked with children most of our lives and my life in some very profound ways. I know what it is to not trust a soul. I know what it is to cringe at the mere thought of being touched, as do all my parts. Collectively we love and have fiercely protected children, both those we knew and know, and others whom we did not.

My parts and my husband are working toward understanding each other. He is now in therapy with us, and while it is very difficult to share some of these things with him, we do it. We did it for him, for me, for them and for all of us.

I'm known as the Queen of Vague, a title that we, especially they, have worked hard to maintain, and they did it extraordinarily well, but now we want more human connection in some instances.

Not one of our roommates ever knew I had DID. They hide well, and I would be gone for very extended periods of time. In truth, I can't even tell you the names of all our roommates.

*

CHRIS ROBIN
Chris was diagnosed with at least
7 personalities in 2013 at age 49

I don't have any children, but as a teacher I am around children all the time. I often wondered what it would have been like to have a child. But most of the time I don't think of myself as the maternal type, and I think I probably would have done more harm than good if I had had a child. I would not have wanted to pass on my issues or problems, and I wouldn't have wanted a child to have to have dealt with my mental issues. It wouldn't have been fair to that child. So most of the time I am grateful that children were not part of my journey.

*
QUINN ROSE
Quinn was diagnosed with 9
personalities in 2016 at age 21

I do not have nor want kids. My boyfriend is very accepting of my alters; he was one of the first ones to know, and he supports me fully. From what he says and from what my alters write in their journals, they like him and trust him somewhat.

*

AYA SAKURA
Aya has been living with 7
personalities since childhood

I do not have any children or a significant other at the moment. My ex-boyfriend did know about my alters, but he couldn't really handle them. He especially had difficulties with Clive being a male alter. You can imagine that led to quite a few awkward situations.

*

FLOSS SCOTT
Floss was diagnosed with at least
4 personalities in 2016 at age 48

I raised three children singlehanded for twenty years, and feel that I did a great job, as people always say my children are a credit to me. It was difficult, especially when I had blackouts and the kids would tell me the stuff I did or said, and I had no memory of it. It was very upsetting. I also lost a lot of family members which caused me to switch more regularly, but at the time I had no clue as to what was wrong with me.

The doctors kept putting me on antidepressants, which made me wild to the point where I had a knife at someone's throat because they were lying to me. I also saw red and beat someone up. When I was younger, I would be pushed to fight and so Miss Aggressive would show. She did fight, and god help anyone who got in her path. She hasn't been out for twenty years, now.

*

KERRYJANE VOTH
Kerryjane was diagnosed with
35 alters in 2013 at age 53

Speaking to the Mother is very triggering, because the Mother holds a lot of trauma memories. So I will try to give a brief overview for her. Having and raising children was very hard physically, emotionally, and spiritually, and also very rewarding, joyful and fun. The Mother had to stay online almost all the time. This was very exhausting. It left little body time for any of the other alters, and there was a lot of fighting that went on internally. Some alters understood that the children's welfare came first and accepted taking a back seat for those years. Other alters didn't understand and just tormented the Mother verbally. Some of the alters were able to come out only when the children were visiting relatives. But it's not clear what went on, because during those years a co-consciousness hadn't developed, and I was experiencing a lot of dissociation.

The children did see evidence of the switching when they would come to the Mother and say she had told them that they could do something, but then she would deny it.

Not all our alters are comfortable around our birth children. And not all the birth children are comfortable around the alters. There is only one mother alter, so if she isn't online the system is not connected to the birth children at all. This has also interfered with keeping attachments to the children as they have grown into adults. My Girl Friend alter, along with Grams, have been able to create a nice relationship with my youngest daughter and her children. It has not been easy to do this. It's taken a lot of trial and error on all our parts. But there is an attachment between the daughter and Mother that has held us together through our learning curves.

*

CHAPTER SEVENTEEN

working with Therapists

Hopefully, the therapist is functioning at a higher level of mental health than is the client, but it is a mistake to take that to mean that the therapist should assume a role of power over the client. Actually, clients are often coping well given what they are coping with. -LYNETTE S. DANYLCHUK

Treatment and therapy of DID can be challenging. A combination of medication and talk therapy is common practice, though it often yields varying results. Have you found clinical therapy helpful?

*

ADRIANNE ALLEN-LANG
Adrianne was diagnosed with 10
personalities in 2015 at age 18

No.

*

GAIL BUSWELL
Gail was diagnosed with 13
personalities in 2002 at age 24

No. Well that was easy to answer!!

*

KATT HART
Katt was diagnosed with hundreds
of personalities in 2011 at age 20

We haven't been lucky enough to find a therapist who can help us so far. We've been in therapy twice and attempted to work with the local mental health teams, but they typically don't know how to work with us, and they turn us away. Our last therapist was with us for eighteen months. She was lovely and helped in some areas, but when it came to DID, she didn't know what to do and didn't know how to approach our past either. We're still looking for someone we can afford to see who's willing to help us.

*

AMELIA JOUBERT
Amelia was diagnosed with 12
personalities in 2013 at age 15

Scarlet answering. Now that we have found a good therapist, therapy is very helpful for us! We have had quite a few different therapists, seven that I can think of. One we stopped seeing because he retired. One didn't believe in DID, one moved away, one was trying to force integration on us when we didn't want it, one was in the residential treatment facility we went to and once we stopped living there we couldn't see her, one felt she didn't have enough experience with DID and recommended we see the therapist we're with now. The therapist we are now with is working on cooperation with us and helping Amelia with her depression, and is a really great man.

Our goal in therapy is cooperation in our system rather than integration, the fusion of all alters into one identity. It is now accepted by many DID specialists that cooperation can be just as effective as integration, sometimes even more so. I trust our therapist, but not everyone in our system does. In fact, I can't think of any therapist whom everyone in our system trusted, and this shouldn't be taken personally, it's to keep us safe.

*

AMANDA LINEBACK
Amanda was diagnosed with hundreds
of personalities in 2013 at age 31

The majority of my experiences with therapists, psychiatrists, and doctors have been terrible. I've been drugged and treated for everything except for the actual cause of my symptoms. The wrong medicine and being misdiagnosed by an experienced therapist is so dangerous. Therapy is hard and it is painful. In order to heal and have better communication, you have to re-experience some trauma. It's hard, and if your life isn't stable it could hurt you badly.

When I started to see Dr. Gable, I knew that she was going to change my life. Dr. Gable treats people with DID, and she definitely found her true calling. I trust her more than I have ever trusted anybody in my life. She tells me she is sorry that I had to go through my abuse, and she would turn back time to protect me if she could. She says it is awful that I had to go through something so scary, and tells me how brave I am. Knowing that someone would go back in time to protect you is a very emotional and powerful experience. I am able to do some of the things I wanted to be able to do because I have been going to therapy.

*

JANE MACDONALD
Jane was diagnosed with 3 personalities in
2014 at age 35, and currently has 6 alters

I find this a difficult question to answer, because I'm in therapy for several mental illnesses in addition to my DID. I have been in therapy most of my life but was diagnosed with DID only two years ago. Even during those two years, I have yet to delve into the trauma history or factors that led to my DID. To date, my current psychiatrist and I focus mostly on other things, such as mood, anxiety, panic, and self-harm. When we discuss my DID it is usually about how often I am switching and how much (or in my case, how little) control I have over the alters. Although at times I feel I have made progress in some areas, such as cutting less or an improved mood, I cannot say for certain if this is the result of finding the right medication or of the talk therapy that I do. At other times I relapse, and any progress I think I've made is lost. I've found therapy to be very cyclical rather than linear in nature. I start out okay, but my functioning gradually decreases until I reach a crisis, and then gradually return to being able to function again.

One of the things I find helpful with my current psychiatrist is that he is accepting and willing to work with all my alters. I'm usually aware when one of them is starting to come out, although I usually blank out after a couple of minutes. However, during those brief moments I know that my psychiatrist is kind and thoughtful, particularly with my youngest alter, who seems to be terrified most of the time. He speaks to her gently, has adapted to using yes or no type questions, because she does not speak. He also makes my appointments during the end of the day on Fridays so there is less noise and people around, as he knows she is often triggered by noise. As frustrated as I get with her coming out, he never judges, and always goes out of his way to be kind to her. He doesn't get frustrated with her when she doesn't speak or is afraid. He asks questions, but if she can't answer he is not demanding in any way. He has even been tolerant and accepting of my more angry alter, even when she apparently tries to self-harm in his office. I know that she does not like or trust him for some reason, but I trust him implicitly and I think my littlest one is starting to trust him as well.

I also like that he speaks to me like an intelligent person, and doesn't patronize me. We talk about theories of DID treatment and come to an agreement together on methods that we want to try as well as ones to avoid. We discuss the merits of certain theories of DID, of their different treatment approaches, and make decisions together. Although he didn't provide much information at first, he now refers me to academic articles and resources on DID to help me further understand my condition. When he prescribes medication, he gives me name of a few to check out and points me to reputable sites to look at their costs and benefits, and then we decide together which ones sound best for me. If they don't work or if I have negative side effects, which I often do, he just does more research and we try another medication. Although I am sure he gets frustrated, as do I, he never shows it. Most of all, I know he cares. I am not just another patient to him. He treats me like a fellow human being, an adult.

Along the way, there have been things in therapy that were not helpful. Many therapists were patronizing, ignored what I was telling them, or simply misdiagnosed and overmedicated me. Although therapy with my current psychiatrist is not perfect, it is a vast improvement from previous therapists.

I do wish certain things had been different, however. First and foremost, when I was initially diagnosed with DID, I wish I had been given information about it or at least told of reputable sources to find such information on my own. I was left to fend for myself, and this meant turning to the internet. Although that can be helpful and have useful information, it can also be very misleading. I was fortunate enough to discover several online DID support groups that I joined, and was able to learn from other members who had been diagnosed for longer and had a much greater understanding of dissociative identity disorder.

I would also have liked to have known that everyone's experience of DID is different. Maybe this is why my psychiatrist didn't give me much information; he didn't want me to be biased and imagine I had some of the textbook symptoms if I didn't actually have them. Unfortunately, in these DID support groups I often ended up comparing myself to others, and could feel very much alone if my symptoms and struggles were different from others in the group.

*

CRYSTALIE MATULEWICZ
Crystalie was diagnosed with dissociative
identity disorder in 2015 at age 29

I've been in and out of therapy since I was fifteen. Most of those instances were not helpful. A lot of that has to do with my diagnosis being wrong for so long. When I first went to therapy, I was diagnosed with bipolar type II. Shortly after, when I told my therapist I was doing things I didn't remember doing, she assumed it was mania and psychosis and changed my diagnosis to bipolar type I. My treatment depended heavily on medications, with a side of mediocre therapy. Of course, the medications didn't help at all because I wasn't truly bipolar. The therapy I received was not good at all; my therapist talked more about herself and her own experiences than I did about mine. I wasn't upset when she left to take another job.

Over the years I continued to receive diagnosis after diagnosis, some of which included major depressive disorder, cyclothymic disorder, generalized anxiety disorder, social anxiety disorder, attachment disorder, ADHD, borderline personality disorder, and, at the age of twenty-eight, posttraumatic stress disorder. It took thirteen years of therapy and treatment before I got a diagnosis that acknowledged my trauma. That wasn't for lack of trying. When I brought up certain issues in therapy, therapists would avoid talking about them. In my second stint in therapy during my late teens, I brought up my struggle with self-injury with my therapist. He wriggled in his chair and changed the topic, and I never brought it up again. When I tried to talk about my struggle with an eating disorder, a different therapist told me that it wasn't an issue that needed to be discussed because I was not underweight. Still yet another therapist told me I was too complex to be treated.

That wasn't the worst of it. I finally revealed in therapy that I had been abused by my mother, and I was met with everything but acceptance. One therapist told me that it wasn't possible. Another therapist told me that I was just confused, that mothers didn't hurt their children like that, and that my mother really loved me. That same therapist told me that I was inappropriately attached to my mother, and handed me a book to read on attachment disorders. I never opened the book. I returned it to the front desk and never went back to that therapist again.

One therapist did believe me, but she didn't have enough experience to understand what was going on with me. I froze during our sessions, and retreated into myself because it was too hard to talk about the trauma in detail. Instead of grounding me or helping me process what was going on, my therapist and I ended up spending most sessions in silence because I wasn't mentally there to engage, and she didn't know how to get me back.

I spent all of 2014 and the first half of 2015 in and out of psychiatric hospitals. I was experiencing consistent flashbacks that left me suicidal. I was also still living with my abuser, which only made my situation worse. At that time, receiving treatment in the hospital was the best option for me although most aren't DID friendly. I was asked several times during hospitalization if I heard voices, and I hesitantly answered no because I knew they would label me psychotic. Hospitals are there to medicate and stabilize, and rarely focus on in-depth diagnosis and treatment. So while my hospital stays kept me safe from abuse, they were damaging in their own way.

I started therapy with my current therapist within a week after I ran away. I knew that she understood me. She wasn't unwilling to talk about trauma. She worked with survivors of abuse, as well as people with DID and PTSD, and she was willing to help me. So I took a final chance at getting help, and it worked, so much so that it is the longest I've ever stayed with the same therapist. I haven't had to give up like I did so many other times before. It's been hard on me financially to continue to go to therapy, but I wasted too many years in therapy that wasn't helpful, and I don't want to lose what I have now. I go without a lot of things because I know that without therapy I would not be functioning right now.

My therapist gets me, as much as someone could understand. She is probably the only person I fully trust, because my ability to trust has been so badly damaged over the decades. I've told my therapist things I would never tell anyone else, things that I would never even have the courage to admit on paper. Some of my parts trust her, but some struggle because of issues we've had in the past with other therapists.

Therapy has been difficult. There are so many things I am having to learn now at thirty years old that I should have learned when I was a child. I've had to learn what feelings are, and that it's okay to have them. I've had to learn how to assert myself. I've had to learn how to ask for what I need. I've had to learn that it's okay to be not okay, and that I don't have to lie to save face anymore.

It's frustrating, because even though I have been going to therapy twice a week for over a year now, it's not enough. People on the outside think I'm doing okay; I go to work, I go to school, I get things done. They don't see how much I am struggling. My therapist sees, but she can do only so much. She can't be there for me every day. I need intensive treatment but I can't afford to miss work. I get stuck for a while until I'm able to pull myself together long enough to make progress before spiraling back down again.

I have so much going on aside from the DID. I'm grieving. I'm grieving the loss of my entire family. I'm grieving the loss of the first twenty-nine years of my life. I'm still struggling with an eating disorder. Every so often my depression has me fall into the black hole of hopelessness, and everything else falls in around me too. I can barely make it through the day. Getting out of bed in the morning seems impossible. It's a lot to deal with. We've had to take steps back and work on stabilization and self-care before we could even approach dealing with trauma and DID.

Processing trauma is something that will never get easier. Some people think it's better to keep the trauma buried and hidden. I tried that for years; it doesn't help me or my parts. Hiding something doesn't mean it doesn't exist. It's like a poison. You can't see it, but it's there, eating away at you from the inside. I break down a lot in therapy. I cry. I panic. I have flashbacks. That's no different than what I was experiencing in my life before and outside of therapy. But now in therapy, I have my therapist there with me, supporting me and helping me process and work through everything. I'm not alone anymore.

*

ALICIA PETTIS
Alicia was diagnosed with 40
personalities in 2015 at age 16

At first I didn't find therapy helpful. All my therapist ever talked about was integration after my diagnosis, and that terrified me and my system. After two or three months of all the protectors and I being persistent, my therapist finally caved and realized that we weren't going to integrate anytime soon. Since then my alter Sophia came out during a therapy appointment and informed my therapist about a lot of things that I don't remember. It helped my therapist get a better insight into my life and my past. Now, who ever wants to talk is the part who comes out, except for the littles; she scares them a lot, so they stay inside. In all honesty, I wish my therapist understood that I don't want to integrate, and when I'm fully in the Dark Room I don't remember what my alters do. She tries hard for me to tell her what they did, but I just can't. Those are the times when I don't believe therapy is the right thing for me.

*

SUNSHINE PURCELL
Denise was diagnosed with 17
personalities in 1995 at age 30

Helpful? Not really. Because while therapists know the term and textbook therapy for DID, they don't see us in front of them. We can talk and describe and ask for things all we want, but if it doesn't fit into the curriculum of their therapy, it's disregarded. For example, I have severe manic depression. My symptoms are only those of bipolar patients, so the antidepressants wouldn't work. My thinking is that depression is depression, it doesn't need a subtitle; just deal with it. Therapists don't know it's all related to having DID, and I didn't know that things like obsessive-compulsive disorder, depersonalization, self-esteem, and behavioral ways also are affected. There shouldn't be a strict guideline. It should be broadened. But it should also not be thought of as untrue or made up. To have DID is way too much work; why would anyone fake it and keep this up for a lifetime?!

Believe me, I fought the diagnosis of DID once I found out, only because I didn't understand, had never heard of it, and was scared. Yet it's simple to understand the mind splitting because something horrific happened to us as a child. It saved our lives, and not coping or knowing how to cope led us to split into more alters, more bad decisions. Thank god for us; we needed a way to work or we wouldn't be alive.

Another thing is that most people who have DID are not violent. Most wouldn't hurt others, because we know what it feels like. I am definitely not a predator even though it was done to me. If anything, I am more protective of my children because of it. I broke the cycle and promised I would never raise my children the way I was raised. They will be better, stronger, independent, and I hope they achieve all they dream about. I don't know if it was enough to raise them that way, because we did live unconventional according to societal standards.

*

ERICKA REEVE
Ericka was diagnosed with over 25
personalities in 2013 at age 26

It has helped immensely. One of my teen parts spent an unbelievable and unimaginable amount of time trying to find help. It took far longer than it should have, and she quite literally tried everything she safely could for us and our personal situations. The most helpful piece is finally knowing why I have massive and empty gaps in my memory, and the knowledge that I am indeed *not* insane.

My therapist is a person, obviously, but fully trust? No, we do not. People are not safe and will eventually flip on you. But that being said, she has helped us for many years now and continues to help. I guess the piece I'd want our therapist to understand better isn't possible. I wish she could understand me, and that I could explain myself better. I've never had some of her conversations with people because I don't really talk to people. I am getting better and have seen some tremendous progress with that, but I find it difficult to express myself in a way ordinary people can comprehend. My brain is not the norm, and I consistently struggle to explain and understand myself, so I can't really expect someone else to have that ability. I suppose we wish we could just place my therapist in my mind for a few minutes, so she can see everything I'm figuring out, where the processes break down, and what we're thinking about at any given moment.

It ranges from having a conversation with them to how I could take apart our television or refrigerator and then repair those items. That's in addition to what it would be like to be a surgeon. I mean if, for example, you needed a mastectomy, which technique would I use, and why? Then would I be able to succeed in removing the necessary tissue? And it just continues from there. At times these things are simultaneously occurring, and then I give myself a wicked migraine, but then I consider how to correct the migraine and what piece of my brain had...

You see a small glimpse of what I mean. This is only the second time we have even attempted to begin to explain the way my brain and thought processes work.

Most people look at you like you've lost your mind. Our therapist did not; she struggled to follow and comprehend how it was that I knew the pieces of our clock and how to dismantle and reassemble them, but reading has always been my escape, so I chalk it up to that. If I go off on a tangent like the one above, I'll likely shrug and laugh uncomfortably and just say I read a lot, or one of them swoops in.

*

CHRIS ROBIN
Chris was diagnosed with at least
7 personalities in 2013 at age 49

I've always firmly believed that God sends the right people into your life for a reason. I've come to learn that God sent me Beth not only to be my life partner, but also to help me and all the parts of me to find some security and stability. For half of my life she provided that to me and I'm very grateful. Now that she's gone, it took some very good friends to convince me to get professional help, and once again God sent me an angel. Therapy has been one of the most difficult things I've had to deal with. It hasn't been easy, but it has been extremely helpful. Learning about how my mind and body function, and learning why I react the way I do and where the parts of me came from has been scary, and yet something that I have known for years that I needed to understand. It takes lots of time and effort, and it can be really easy to walk away from and avoid, but I also know that I wouldn't be here if it weren't for my therapist. I would have taken my life to not go through this living hell, but I am learning that life might be worth going on.

I heard many horror stories of people not being able to find the right kind of therapy or therapist, but I was one of the lucky ones who found the right person who wanted to help me. I also know that I have to give myself some credit for persisting and continuing to go to therapy even when I know that it's hard. Taking the time to make myself a priority and to help myself was the first step to learning to get to know all the parts of me.

*

QUINN ROSE
Quinn was diagnosed with 9
personalities in 2016 at age 21

I haven't gone for a while. Life and money have gotten in the way, but I hope it will help.

*

AYA SAKURA
Aya has been living with 7
personalities since childhood

Personally, I am still in the stage of figuring out what I want to gain from therapy. I have therapy now to get more confident and to be more in touch with myself emotionally. The problem I face is that I have to get in touch with Brianna, since she knows most about my emotions. But she's not very willing to cooperate. I am very scared of talking to my current therapist about my alters, so I avoid that subject. I don't make very much progress at the moment, but I do learn very much from my sessions, and it helps me to better recognize problems and problematic patterns.

*

FLOSS SCOTT
Floss was diagnosed with at least
4 personalities in 2016 at age 48

Since I've been diagnosed and getting help in coming to terms with all my diagnoses, I'm understanding myself better and everything in my life now has a meaning. So far the help I am getting has been good, but I do fear the system because it has let me down before. It took six years for them to diagnose me with DID.

*

KERRYJANE VOTH
Kerryjane was diagnosed with
35 alters in 2013 at age 53

Yes, we have found therapy to be a lifeline to functioning in this body and to being able to manage living in the outside world independently. Therapy has given us an education in everything about DID and PTSD. We've learned how the brain works before and after trauma, how the vagus nerve reacts to stressors, and how all this translates into how humans process trauma and how it affects consciousness.

Therapy has provided the experience of attachment so that our system can know what healthy attachment is supposed to feel and look like within a close and safe relationship. Therapy has helped the body de-traumatize the physical memory feelings, and has helped to lessen the guilt and shame of being abused. Many parts of our system do trust our therapist, as well as many parts who still don't trust. There is no way to hurry this process along, either. The best we can do is to talk to the system as a whole, reminding everyone of the trust that has been developed so far, and to keep an open and curious mind.

I wish my therapist were able to go inside with me so she could be part of the group discussions that go on. As it is, because there is only one body between us all, we have to take turns speaking. This causes a lot of frustration and exhaustion, and some parts never get a turn to speak. We also wish that our therapist could know who is speaking to her, and acknowledge them by name. If you have ever been treated like you are invisible by another human being, then you will know how a lot of our alters feel when we are speaking to you but you aren't speaking to us. You think you are speaking to someone else. It can feel very rejecting and disrespectful.

*

May
BY SUNSHINE

May today there be peace within.

May you trust that you are

exactly where you are meant to be.

May you not forget the infinite possibilities that are

born of faith in yourself and others.

May you use the gifts that you have received,

And pass on the love that has been given to you.

May you be content with yourself just the way you are.

Let this knowledge settle into your bones, and allow

your soul the freedom to sing, dance, praise and love.

It is there for each and every one of us.

*

CHAPTER EIGHTEEN

Explaining our uniqueness

Here we are, unique, eternal aspects of consciousness with an infinity of potential. -DAVID ICKE

Whether one has two alters or many, it remains challenging for the outside world to understand the uniqueness of living with different parts, alters, identities, and personalities. What is the best way to explain how it feels to have numerous parts who each hold different memories and different preferences sharing the same body?

*

ADRIANNE ALLEN-LANG
Adrianne was diagnosed with 10
personalities in 2015 at age 18

It feels like you're in a room with six-plus TVs going at once. Two are playing reality TV, two are playing completely different movies, one is blasting music, and the other is watching the cooking channel. It's cramped, noisy and loud, but most days I wouldn't change it even if I could.

*

GAIL BUSWELL
Gail was diagnosed with 13
personalities in 2002 at age 24

To me, DID means feeling lost. Lost in time, time that is just billowing and sometimes spits me out. It is not knowing whether I will remember or experience the complete day and simple tasks like feeding the fish, cleaning, and spending time with friends. It lacks context, orientation, understanding and knowledge. It is having pictures of horrible scenes in front of my eyes, and immense pain both physical and emotional—and being confronted with pain and suffering that feels so strange and horrifying. It is disconnection, being disconnected to the body and my surroundings. It is body dysmorphia. On the other side, it means learning a lot about other opinions and reactions and attitude, and realizing how messed up this world can be.

*

KATT HART
Katt was diagnosed with hundreds
of personalities in 2011 at age 20

The best way I can describe what it's like to have DID is that the body we live in is a car or bus, and multiple people drive it around and do what they like with it. Others around you always call you by the car's name. It's like calling someone Mercedes instead of calling him John. It's being unrecognized and ignored by most people around you, or people getting confused that you aren't the car itself, that you're the driver and you have a name. You don't even look like the car. You were born at a different time as the car, so why does everyone keep repeating that mistake?

The car goes through having modifications done to it without the other drivers knowing. That's absolutely irritating, and causes arguments. Why would someone put that paint on the car, and throw out the paint I used? They get into accidents all the time. The car is already a bit beaten up, and now some idiot is driving who keeps causing more damage! Also, the car is hard to repair. Help isn't always available, or maybe you can't afford the help, so a lot of that work is done by the drivers who probably don't know what they're doing and could make it worse.

Some drivers go out in the car to buy loads of stuff you don't need, and spend most, if not all, the money that you have to share. Some even invite other people to hang out near your car who you don't know. Can you trust that person, or will they do something to damage the car too? Someone took the car out a week ago, and now someone else hasn't been able to leave the house since. What are they doing with the car, and why do they need it for so long? All you want is for the current driver to contact you to let you know that the car's okay, and what's been happening for the last week.

There are so many options that can happen. If you can imagine sharing your car with a load of other people and think of any other situation that could happen, then it's probably similar to how we would describe living with DID. It's such a pain, and half the time you don't have control over what's happening with your car but you can't do anything about it. You just have to learn to cooperate with the other drivers, figure out what everyone needs, and maybe get a schedule if you think you need one. You're stuck with sharing it, so you might as well learn to get along with one another.

*

AMELIA JOUBERT
Amelia was diagnosed with 12
personalities in 2013 at age 15

Scarlet answering. When we say we share a body with other people, that's exactly what we mean. It's not one person acting like different people; we are literally different people and would appreciate being treated as such. Technically, we are all parts of a whole, but think about it this way: you wouldn't call Texas and New Jersey the same state just because they are both part of the United States. Alters are parts of a whole, yet completely different. Even if alters are similar, that doesn't mean they are the same. North Carolina and South Carolina may be similar and close in proximity, but that doesn't make them the same state.

*

AMANDA LINEBACK
Amanda was diagnosed with hundreds
of personalities in 2013 at age 31

Imagine that your head space is a huge auditorium. It is dark in the auditorium, so you can't see anything but you can hear other people talking. When there are triggers, flashlights are turned on by some people and sometimes the whole auditorium lights up. In that auditorium there are many kinds of people. We don't know each other, and sometimes we don't like each other. When it's time to eat, the entire group gets to pick one thing and it has to be unanimous. The fighting, contemplating, and discussing that goes on in order to get the group to make a decision is what is going on in my head—at all times of the day—regarding every single aspect of my life.

*

JANE MACDONALD
Jane was diagnosed with 3 personalities in
2014 at age 35, and currently has 6 alters

The best way I've heard DID explained is to liken it to driving a car. Sometimes you're the driver and in full control, making all the decisions about where to go and what to do, and other personalities are the passengers. Other times, you're a passenger and someone else is driving. You can see what is going on and you're aware of what he or she is doing, and you can grab the steering wheel to avert disaster if needed.

Sometimes you're in the backseat and have minimal awareness of what is going on. You can try to talk to the personality who is driving, and influence him or her, but ultimately have very little control over what is going on. Sometimes you are in the trunk. You cannot hear or see or influence what is going on. You have no control whatsoever, and can only go along for the ride and try to figure things out later.

People need to know that we don't always have control of who is driving, or for how long. Some have developed systems of communication with their other personalities, and are able to exert greater influence. Unfortunately, not all situations are like this. Many of us are left out of the decision-making process, and when an alter decides it's their turn to drive, there is little we can do to prevent the alter from taking over.

*

CRYSTALIE MATULEWICZ
Crystalie was diagnosed with dissociative
identity disorder in 2015 at age 29

It doesn't always feel the same. Some days I feel like a normal singleton. I feel in control of myself. There is quiet in my mind. There is peace in my body. Some days I wake up and feel like I just walked into a classroom with thirty unsupervised kindergartners, except the classroom is in my head and the kindergartners are my younger parts vying for attention. Some days it feels like I'm sitting back and watching a movie, except the movie is my life and my parts are the actors. I can't control what's happening, I can only sit back and watch it all unfold. It's my movie, but I'm not acting in it. It's my life, but I'm not living it.

Sharing a body is like sharing a car. Sometimes I'm the driver behind the wheel, in control of where I'm go and my parts are all in back. Okay, perhaps a bus is more appropriate for this visual; squishing all my parts into the back of a car sounds. When one of my parts decides it's his or her turn to drive, he or she takes the wheel and I go to the back of the bus. I'm still there, I'm just not in control.

Sometimes, a part decides he or she wants to drive but I don't want to give up control. My part may try to grab the wheel, and I lose control for a moment until I grab the wheel right back again. That part then becomes a backseat driver, giving me directions and making decisions on where he or she thinks I should go, and what I should do. They are not in full control, but their presence is certainly known, whether it's wanted or not.

That bus is our body. We are always inside. We are always together. But control is shared by who is at the wheel, and a license is never required to drive.

*

ALICIA PETTIS
Alicia was diagnosed with 40
personalities in 2015 at age 16

I explain having alters like this. Imagine going to sleep, and in your dreams there are people. Those people are the alters. Now what if your body begins to sleepwalk and sleep talk? You're still dreaming, but your body is doing other things, and telling people to call you by a different name, but it's not your name. When you wake up, you find new people in your phone contacts, you're in a new house, or you have new clothes. Sometimes you can hear or see the people from your dream, except this time you're not sleeping, you're in control of your own body.

When people knows someone has DID, I want them to call the alters by the correct names. My alters know that sometimes it's hard for someone to grasp the understanding that it's not the host, but it also irritates them to have to answer to my name. When someone gets his or her name right, it fills them with joy.

*

SUNSHINE PURCELL
Denise was diagnosed with 17
personalities in 1995 at age 30

There is constant chatter or noise in my head. It never stops. We are always on alert. We've always had to be aware of our surroundings in order to survive. We are not crazy, and most who live with DID are not violent. We live in a world that we had no choice in. We live with the consequences that others have put on us. We are rational in all we do for the irrational situation we were exposed to. This is real life for us. We struggle and we question and we are different. But aren't we all different? People with DID are just to the extreme, that's all.

*

ERICKA REEVE
Ericka was diagnosed with over 25
personalities in 2013 at age 26

So you're driving a car, all is well and good, and suddenly it's five months later and you find yourself at the beach. It feels dream-like, almost a dizziness and floating. And it depends on the part. It's like driving a car, and kids or other passengers are constantly arguing or asking repeated questions like "Are we there yet?" There's playing and then crying. Singing and then screaming. Trying to speak and no words come out. It can be terrifying, but now I find comfort in even my most vocal and mean (protective, not mean) parts.

As a collective, we very much want people to understand that we spent my life simply trying to survive. We are not dangerous or evil or crazy. I and we want to live. We are no longer satisfied with the bare minimum, survival; now, we want to actually live.

*

CHRIS ROBIN
Chris was diagnosed with at least
7 personalities in 2013 at age 49

I wish I knew a way to explain it. But then again, the only ones who need to know are the people who live with and love us for who we are, and still want to love us. Everybody else is probably satisfied with the part of me they interact with, or they wouldn't be around. It's the easiest way to know who true friends, family, and lovers really are. They are the ones who stick around even when they see you switch. They are okay with you being several parts and switching, and don't need a definition or an explanation.

Those who accept us for who we are, rather than just tolerate us, are the only ones to whom I feel like I want to explain to, but it's not a conversation I've been able to have with anyone except my therapist. Maybe this book will provide an opportunity to have someone learn about DID, and it will open the conversation about what is going on in my head. The scariest thought in my world is that someone close to me would no longer accept me if they knew I had DID, or would treat me differently because of it. That's why I haven't told anyone.

*

QUINN ROSE
Quinn was diagnosed with 9
personalities in 2016 at age 21

It's like you never truly know who you are. You have other things working against you. You may have people supporting you, but always feel like a burden and constantly want to run away to live in solitude.

*

AYA SAKURA
Aya has been living with 7
personalities since childhood

I think the best way of explaining how it feels to have alters sharing the same body to outsiders is using the analogy of a car. Imagine your body as a car. If you have the wheel, then you control the body. If you are in the passenger seat, you get the same sensory input as if you have the wheel, but you can't control the body, though you can sometimes get your hand on the wheel and influence the way of driving. If you're in the back seat, you get less sensory input, like only the details or an outline of what's going on. If you're in the trunk, you don't know what's going on; it's almost like being unconscious, or being in a black space of nothingness.

Now imagine there are a number of strangers in the same car. You have the wheel and are trying to get where you want to go, even though there are others in the car who are in the back, some in the trunk, and some in the passenger seat. Everyone wants to go someplace else, everyone has other ideas of how to drive, and everyone has an idea of what the car should look like. Some just tell you where to drive to, some try to argue with you, others try to take over the wheel, a few don't care, even if the car crashes, but only one of you can get his or her way.

If you get lucky, everyone wants to go to the same place, and then you can cooperate and drive to your destination together. This is kind of how it feels to have alters. And it's hard.

*
FLOSS SCOTT
Floss was diagnosed with at least
4 personalities in 2016 at age 48

I really haven't spoken to anyone outside of the professionals about what it's like. My children have lived with me all their lives, so to them, I'm just Mom, and this is how I'm made. My sisters said they always knew I had different personalities, so this is who they know, and it makes no difference to them. I haven't quite thought of how I would tell other people. To be honest, I won't tell anyone unless I really have to. This is me. Yes, I have other versions of me sharing my body, and I'm proud that I am who I am.

*

KERRYJANE VOTH
Kerryjane was diagnosed with
35 alters in 2013 at age 53

I think the best way that I have found to explain DID is to approach it from a common experience. I like to start at the beginning, and give the example of how every child starts out in life with unintegrated consciousness. As we grow, we start to integrate between the ages of six and nine. This is a very normal development, and as long as a child is not traumatized, this integration will take place naturally. I was traumatized sometime before that age, and didn't develop integrated consciousness. Over the years, each of my parts continued to develop individually. This individuality was maintained through amnesia between each part.

*

Forever to Sleep
BY SUNSHINE

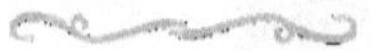

I close my eyes once more and hope the ugliness disappears,
only to find again opened eyes welt up with tears.
I have tried so hard to forget the images of my past
but the door never remains locked and the chains never last.
Memories dancing freely around and around in my head
echoing like rolls of thunder, never hearing what they've said.
Lost in mass confusion, feeling reality slip away;
my nights have become forever long
never seeing the light of day.
My feelings are not felt, they are lost inside this hole
and the spirit that once gave light
lives no longer within my soul.
My mind has dulled all senses, while my body feels no pain.
There are cuts beneath the surface
leaving scars within my brain.
The color of my eyes, the brightness that once was there
has become cold black pools of emptiness
that holds an empty stare.
What is it that I've been fighting, fighting to survive
and how long must this guard stay up before I feel alive.
My days are filled with chaos, as I scatter from room to room;
the simple things in life once that brought much pleasure
seem forever an impending doom.
Such a deep aching inside, silently it weeps
knowing the utter truth: nothing is for keeps.
Fragmented, jagged edges, like glass that has been shattered
desperately searching for the pieces,
some lost but mostly scattered.
I feel I have no more strength; I feel frail and I feel weak.
The innocence that was taken
is my dream I forever seek.
I will not tell my ugly secrets for they are buried oh so deep
only to awaken while the world outside is asleep.
I close my tired eyes once more,
praying closed that they will stay
as my breath I take of "this kind of life" I wish
quietly slips away.

CHAPTER NINETEEN

Finding a Silver Lining

I am made of all the things that this world
couldn't take from me. -RUDY FRANSISCO

Despite the hand that life dealt, some are determined to remain hopeful that a sliver of light can be found in the darkness, a silver lining of some sort. It's human resiliency at its finest. Have you discovered a silver lining from your journey with DID?

*

ADRIANNE ALLEN-LANG
Adrianne was diagnosed with 10
personalities in 2015 at age 18

Even when I feel lonely, I'm never alone.

*

GAIL BUSWELL
Gail was diagnosed with 13
personalities in 2002 at age 24

Maybe one silver lining is if life gets too much, someone else will always be there to take over.

*

KATT HART
Katt was diagnosed with hundreds
of personalities in 2011 at age 20

There's absolutely a silver lining. We alters have each other, we have so many friends and perspectives and skills within one body but many people. Of course it isn't the same as having friends outside our own body, but it's one of the things that keeps us going. We get to experience so many different things, because so many different people enjoy doing things. We learn more because different people have different interests. We grow as a big group of people every day, and that's an incredible thing to us.

*

SUNSHINE PURCELL
Denise was diagnosed with 17
personalities in 1995 at age 30

The silver lining for me is that I have a whole bunch of others inside of me willing and able to love. I am kind and compassionate and care about others who struggle with life. My mind is genius for developing a way that allowed me to survive what happened to me. I'm a survivor, but I am not defined by what I have. That is only part of it. I have gifts and talents that I am grateful for.

*

ERICKA REEVE
Ericka was diagnosed with over 25
personalities in 2013 at age 26

I suppose the big easy response to a question about a silver lining would be that I'm still alive. Additionally though, Minny tends to do my dishes and, when she can, the laundry and cleaning. Who would want to do dishes? (lol)

*

FLOSS SCOTT
Floss was diagnosed with at least
4 personalities in 2016 at age 48

The silver lining to this is that not everybody out there is as shallow and evil as the man I married. There are good, decent people out there, and many who live with DID have successful relationships and marriages.

*

Inside
BY SUNSHINE

Look deep inside my heart and tell me what I feel,

for sometimes I do not know if what I feel is real.

Look deep into my eyes, the place I like to hide

where everything I need to feel safe, is locked up tight inside.

I ask you when I cry, to let my tears fall where they may,

for the tears may be my words, the words I cannot say.

I beg you not to be angry with me when I cannot speak,

when my voice will only whisper, and comfort is what I seek.

I know it sounds never-ending, the sadness that you hear,

but it's the caring and you listening that helps me with my fear.

I am so very sorry that you are burdened with my past,

it hurts me that that I cannot tell you how long this all will last.

For you are the first, the only one who's asked

"Why do you hurt? What pains have you masked?"

Just know that I have never given

all of me to anyone including you,

for in that comes great trust,

and a love that should be true.

*

CHAPTER TWENTY

Walking the Journey

I don't want my pain and struggle to make me a victim. I want my battle to make me someone else's hero. -ANONYMOUS

Every journey is unique as a fingerprint, for we experience different beliefs, desires, needs, and often walk different roads. Though we may not see anyone else on the path, we are never truly alone, for more walk behind, beside, and in front of us. In this chapter lies the answers to the final question: What would you like the world to know about your mental illness journey?

*

ADRIANNE ALLEN-LANG
Adrianne was diagnosed with 10
personalities in 2015 at age 18

Dissociative identity disorder is not scary. We are loving, caring people who have been through hell and back within our lives, and this is how we cope. We are just extra special and there are more of us to love and be loved!

*

GAIL BUSWELL
Gail was diagnosed with 13
personalities in 2002 at age 24

It isn't fun. It isn't fake. It isn't a show, and it's hard work

*

KATT HART
Katt was diagnosed with hundreds
of personalities in 2011 at age 20

Living with DID is difficult and confusing. Nothing is straight forward, and it's scary having to get to know all these others who live in the same body, especially knowing that they could hold horrible memories. Each person with DID is different. Each has a different way to cope and different goals. It's so important to get to know those things about every person with DID. But be careful not to push them; let them take things at a pace that feels comfortable.

They may not want their alters acknowledged as different people, or they may want to be acknowledged as separate people, like we do. They may want to integrate, or they may want to stay multiple, or even a mixture of the two by integrating some. Each of these choices is very personal, and no choice is wrong. It's so important to treat someone with DID as he or she wants and needs to be treated.

It's very important to remember that there's probably going to be alters who will cause damage. They'll hurt the other alters, or even outsiders, and they'll self-harm or sabotage good things. But these alters should never be rejected or talked about horribly. We guarantee you that they think they're doing the right thing. They've been taught somehow that this is the way to act because it might get them less hurt, or they've been told that certain people or alters deserve it. You have to work with these alters, help them feel human and cared for, rather than treating them like monsters. Usually if you treat people as if they're bad, they'll show you just how bad they can be. But if you show them kindness and love, they may begin to rethink how they've been acting. This will be an ongoing battle, but it's worth all the work that's put into it.

Whether you have DID or not, always treat alters with respect and don't treat them like horrible symptoms that need to leave. It'll do more harm than good in the end. Every alter deserves to be heard and deserves a chance to experience nice, normal things outside of the trauma.

*

AMELIA JOUBERT
Amelia was diagnosed with 12
personalities in 2013 at age 15

I want the world to know that DID doesn't make us dangerous. Statistically, we are no more likely to commit a crime than someone without DID. We are able to function pretty well. Yes, we do have struggles, but I'm sure singlets (non-multiples) also have struggles; ours are just a little different. Just because we function and live our lives a bit differently than you doesn't make it any better or worse. We can be, and many of us are, productive members of society! Signing off, Amelia, Scarlet, and the rest of the labyrinth system!

*

AMANDA LINEBACK
Amanda was diagnosed with hundreds
of personalities in 2013 at age 31

I am Amanda June Lineback and I have dissociative identity disorder.

I want to change the way the world looks at dissociative identity disorder. When people talk about a person who has DID, I want my face and my life to come to their minds. I want to make treatment available that doesn't traumatize us even more when we are trying to get help.

The people who have known me my entire life have never been told that I am a multiple. If I have to go to the doctor, I keep the fact that I am a multiple hidden. People are afraid of things they don't know much about, especially if it is stigmatized to be something it is not. People with DID are some of the most empathetic, loving, sweet, individuals that I know. Triggers terrify us and we spend most of our lives running from them. Dissociative identity disorder is the reason why I am alive today. I am thankful and love everyone inside. They are my family and they have never let me down.

*

JANE MACDONALD
Jane was diagnosed with 3 personalities in
2014 at age 35, and currently has 6 alters

I want people to know that not everyone's experience of DID is the same. If you meet someone and are fortunate enough for that person to share with you that he or she has DID, please don't judge the person based on your preconceptions of what DID is. Don't compare them with others you may know who have DID. Especially don't assume it's the same as it's often depicted in a novel or movie or in the media. We are all unique individuals. Though we may share a diagnosis, we are just like you; with our own unique struggles and strengths.

People with DID are like anyone else with a medical disorder, or really anyone at all; we are all unique. No one experiences any illness exactly the same way. We may have similar symptoms such as loss of time, the presence of other personalities, etc., but please do not compare us, and do not expect us to be just like Tara from the show "United States of Tara," or the movie "Sybil."

Some have an elaborate inside world, with places where our other personalities go when they are not fronting. Others, like myself, do not. Some people have two alters, while others have hundreds. Some have alters with different genders, race, sexual orientation, religion, cultures, and sometimes even species. Some people have animal or half-animal alters. Please do not judge us by how well we fit into your idea of what DID is. This is something I wish for the psychiatric community in particular, to recognize that not everyone's symptoms and experiences fit into these nice little boxes in the DSM-V or the ones previous to it. Sometimes you need to think out of the box, or forget the box altogether and just listen to what people are telling you they experience.

If someone chooses to tell you he or she has DID, please realize that they are trusting you not to judge or condemn them for who they are. Please realize that it is very difficult for us to share this diagnosis with others, even mental health professionals, because it is still so highly stigmatized, and because of the inaccuracies that exist in the media. We are taking a great risk by telling others about our condition, and the last thing we need is to be judged, compared, ridiculed, or made to feel bad. Please be thankful that we are able to share our struggle with you, and be open to listening to what our experience is like. We may not want to share a lot with you, or we may feel safe enough to tell you a great deal about it. Please listen with open ears, and open heart, and an open mind.

Please also know that there is no cure for DID. Indeed, many of us do not wish to be free of our other personalities. Some of us work toward integrating so that all our personalities merge and become one. Others, however, find this idea upsetting, and cherish their alters as invaluable parts of themselves whom they could not imagine living without. Some people don't see DID as a form of mental illness at all, just as a different way of living and experiencing the world. Please do not be quick to label all of us as ill, or as having a disorder. Just realize that this is how we are, usually due to childhood trauma. Please accept us and be willing to learn about our experiences, should we feel comfortable enough to share them with you.

*

CRYSTALIE MATULEWICZ
Crystalie was diagnosed with dissociative
identity disorder in 2015 at age 29

We are not the people with multiple personalities you see on TV crime shows and in the movies. Most times those portrayals are grossly inaccurate. People living with DID are not murderers or serial killers. We are no more likely to be violent than any non-DID person. In fact, many of us find any kind of violence appalling because we experienced forms of violence in our early lives.

I am not dangerous. The only person I hurt is myself. I know what it's like to be in tremendous pain. I wouldn't put another human being through that. I avoided hurting the very people responsible for my trauma, the very people who many believe deserve to be hurt. I just want to live my life, our life, in the safest way possible.

I am capable. Just because I have DID, and just because I have mental illness, does not mean I am not able to do things. I've excelled academically my whole life. I'm highly intelligent. I've achieved things that many non-DID people could not achieve. I am a writer. I've created things. Don't let my diagnosis get in the way of that.

I want the world to understand that I am not always me. Yes, I am thirty. But many times I am also five, six, seven, eight, ten, twelve, or fifteen. My body doesn't change, but my mind does. You may call me a baby because you see me crying or throwing a tantrum, but sometimes I am a child. You may think I'm acting like an angst-filled teenager. That's because sometimes I *am* an angst-filled teenager.

My parts aren't always like the thirty-year-old me. They think like the ages they are. They like the things that they like, because they are their own people. My five-year-old part likes dinosaurs and animal games. He doesn't understand adult language like I do. My six-year-old part likes doggies and flowers. She has no interest in statistical analysis like I do. My twelve-year-old part likes the color purple and enjoys reading. I like the color blue and find reading to be difficult. We may share the same body, but we are all individuals and deserve to be treated like individuals.

I don't expect people to understand my fear, but I wish they wouldn't judge it. Most people can't understand why I am still so scared of my mother. They assume I am being dramatic. I am not. The fear is real, and is experienced by my parts and me every day of our lives. When you've been badly traumatized, that fear doesn't just go away once you leave the trauma. It still lives inside you.

I want people to know that I can't move on. I can't just get over it. And I can't let it go. My parts and I relive the trauma over and over again. As much as I try to tell my parts that we are safe, as much as I try to show them the good in the world, something triggers us and sets us back. I can't just get over my DID. There is no medication that will make it go away. I work hard in therapy, but I will never be whole.

I can't just forget what was done to me. It has impacted every aspect of my life. I can't knock on a door without remembering the terrible things that existed behind a door when I was younger. I can't take a shower without panicking. I can't eat a meal without determining whether or not I deserve to eat that day. I can't go to sleep at night without fearing that my mother will come into my room and hurt me. Bathing, eating, sleeping…these are all things most people do every day without thinking about it. But I can't do that. I have to work hard just to make it through the day, because life is a constant reminder of what we've been through.

I am learning the things I should have learned in childhood. I am learning how to feel. I am learning how to be assertive. I am learning how to communicate with people using my words. I am learning independence. I am learning how to trust. I am constantly learning. I need support. I need understanding. I don't need judgment.

I spent most of my life in hiding; I didn't have much of a choice. But now I have choices. I made the decision to be open about my diagnosis because I didn't want to hide anymore. I didn't want to feel ashamed of who I was, who we were. I wanted others with DID to know that they don't have to feel ashamed, either.

We didn't choose this disorder. We developed it because it was the only way to survive. And we are surviving.

*

ALICIA PETTIS
Alicia was diagnosed with 40
personalities in 2015 at age 16

Living with DID is both difficult and easy. Having to explain to friends, family, and even teachers that you're a multiple isn't exactly something that's the easiest fly-by in the world. It's difficult, and when I did so, my family looked at me with disgust.

It's also hard for friends to understand what dissociating is like. Many of my friends will leave me by myself when I begin to dissociate, because they don't know how to help. They try the best they can, but they don't know how it feels and they don't know what to say. If someone is beginning to dissociate in front of you, ask the person what is okay for you to do. Is it okay for you to hold them? Is it okay for you to talk to them? Is it okay for them to bring an animal? But don't ask while they're dissociating; wait until they're not. I wouldn't want to be overloaded with questions while trying to battle with reality.

All in all, be kind to those with DID. They've seen things and gone through so much that they need those alters. We need our multiplicity.

*

SUNSHINE PURCELL
Denise was diagnosed with 17
personalities in 1995 at age 30

Every day is a new day, a new opportunity, a new struggle. We can't help having trigger times, nightmares, or flashbacks. We are doing the best we can with what we have to work with. We are, and can be, capable people. We have jobs if we can handle them, and we can raise children who are smart and independent.

We aren't to be feared. We had our lives and innocence taken from us, but we are not stupid or need to be feared. Most times it's just a matter of trust and loyalty. That's something we didn't have, so it's very important to have these in any of our relationships.

Don't mess with us, because it can destroy us more than you think. Just give us a chance; you won't be sorry, or bored. And it's possible to have a happy life.

*

ERICKA REEVE
Ericka was diagnosed with over 25
personalities in 2013 at age 26

First and foremost, DID looks different for everyone. It can be terrifying, unnerving, horrific, silly, loud, enjoyable (at times) and exceptionally lonely. People with DID, people like us, live with each other. We're very different people in most instances, but we want to live as people, meaning that we want acknowledgment and respect. We are not freaks, and we're not evil or malicious. Mischievous, you bet, but we do seek out interactions with no intent to harm.

We want to live our life, our lives, and we want understanding and acceptance. I want people to know that my parts are not demon possession. Religion is a piece of our trauma, and it shouldn't have been that way. My life did not need to become *our* life, and it sure as s*** did not need to become what it was. We want people to realize that some of my parts are exceptionally talented writers (not so much the case for me, so I apologize, lol). Others are amazing at watercolor painting, some excel in math, and others have studied world religions to protect and gain information. Additionally, DID at its core is about survival. All of us, including everyone in this book, did that—we survived. Now I would imagine that we very much want to live.

"Normal is illusion. What is normal for the spider is chaos for the fly." —Morticia Addams. This quote has stuck with us for a very long time. I want to find my own definition of normal. DID isn't fun when you've no idea what is happening and why. It is not a joke, a Halloween costume or make-believe.

It comes along with many other disorders in many instances. My parts struggle with some of their own individual health problems. We want people to know that basic human kindness goes a long, long way. If you or someone you know or care about is struggling, be there without judgment. Someone asking why when we were young could have drastically altered my life for the better. If you see something, say something, and just be there.

*

CHRIS ROBIN
Chris was diagnosed with at least
7 personalities in 2013 at age 49

I just want to live in a world that feels safe, truly values diversity, and understands that all people, even people with DID, have worth. Living is hard, and living with DID is hard. But all the parts of me want to live in a world without loneliness, without fear for our safety, and want to find love.

We know all of us are different, and our uniqueness is what makes this world a special place to be. I just want people to know that even though I might be different, and seem like I have it all together and am confident and know what I'm doing in some situations, doesn't mean that I have it together in other situations. Inside me is a scared child who just wants someone to love her and hold her hand, and a rebellious young man who is willing to die for a cause, and a bunch of cute cuddly parts who love to play, laugh and love freely. If you don't see that part of me, it's because we put up walls to protect ourselves. We just need patience and time to get comfortable with you, and see if you are willing to stick around.

*

QUINN ROSE
Quinn was diagnosed with 9
personalities in 2016 at age 21

It's hard. DID is not to be romanticized about, nor is it to be feared. It's just survival. I only just now learned that I have this, but I'm not as scared as I was not knowing. Knowing that you can be a different person at any time in front of anyone is not fun. It can ruin friendships, relationships, family. Be careful what you say or do to us, because it can change our lives forever. It can change and alter who they are. I am We, and eventually I will know who We are.

*

AYA SAKURA
Aya has been living with 7
personalities since childhood

I want the world to know that I'm still able to function normally even with my system. Because of my system, I'm able to function normally. Otherwise I would have broken down a long time ago. We really liked writing all this down. Clive helped me write this. I got demotivated after quickly and shortly answering the questions, but he got me back on track and wrote down huge parts of my (our) journey for this project. It helped me understand my condition a bit better and made us write down our story (finally), and I am really thankful for this project.

For all the others struggling with DID, you are not alone. You are not fighting this battle alone. There are more of us, and we are all valid.

*

FLOSS SCOTT
Floss was diagnosed with at least
4 personalities in 2016 at age 48

My life had been very confusing before I learned I had DID. Once I was diagnosed and did my research, my whole life fell into context. I understood all the things I was so confused about. This has taken a huge weight off my shoulders, and the worry as to why I had had so many blackouts. As long as I have the support of my children I will be happy. They are the ones who have seen all my different alters, and they know how to deal with each of me.

Sometimes I'm on my own and feel lonely and isolated, but I've learned how to deal with it. I do what works for me; I do positive things like sewing and crafts. I enjoy this, and it takes me back to my happy place where I can't get hurt. I feel safe. This is my Happy Safe Place. I know and understand that we all have different experiences and levels with DID. I still need to research it more. I totally feel for all who are living with DID.

I would say to the world:

Don't look at me differently today than you did yesterday, now that you know I have DID.

Be sympathetic instead of running away.

Look up to us, instead of looking down on us, as we are dealing with a heavier load than you.

Face us and embrace us instead of facing away and turning your back on us.

Empathy goes a long way, and sometimes we need that too.

Think before you speak.

Remember, we all have some form of baggage; it's just that we have a little bit more.

I have a body and mind just like you, only a few people are sharing mine.

DID isn't going to destroy me; it's making me stronger.

*

KERRYJANE VOTH
Kerryjane was diagnosed with
35 alters in 2013 at age 53

I would like the world to know that living with DID can be wonderfully exciting. There is always something new happening, like new ideas, thoughts, feelings, activities, and interests. Living with DID is like being part of a collective: you are never alone. DID provides the most amazing experiences in empathy. We can see multiple points of view in any situation.

*

Struggling
BY SUNSHINE

Struggling for control, chaos at every end

To eat or not eat, the messages always send.

Voices in my head fighting between the two

not about being selfish, no more about being you.

TV, magazines and society all have set the stage

creating a horrific monster full of despair and rage.

Ready to do for others, eager to always please

hiding away the pain while guilt is eager to seize.

Put on your face and hide and all seems just fine

no one ever knowing, you're walking a very thin line.

You can't look in the mirror afraid of what you will see

just a faint resemblance, the reflection that's there was me.

Wasting away to nothing, growing smaller day by day

with no possible way to find me, then I should feel okay.

You know what you are doing. You know it's just not right,

but the fear is overwhelming and your much too tired to fight.

If we all could stand together and fight to be free,

one day our voices would echo

"It's all right to just be me."

*

MEET THE WRITERS

Who are we - DID
BY the system known as Kerryjane Voth
September 22, 2016

. . . we are like flickering
sparkles of sunshine
on the water.

Undulating between
cosciousness,
unconsciousness
and coconsciousness...

a never ending shifting
of knowledge,
skill and ability.

With waves of derealizing
and depersonalizing
and then dissociating...

That break upon the sands
of life
that keep wearing off
our rough edges . . .

*

*

ADRIANNE ALLEN-LANG
Adrianne was diagnosed with 10
personalities in 2015 at age 18

Adrianne Allen-Lang was born in a small town in New South Wales, Australia. Her parents split when she was two years old, and then her mother moved her and her younger brother to the city when Adrianne was five. After moving fourteen hours away at age fourteen to escape 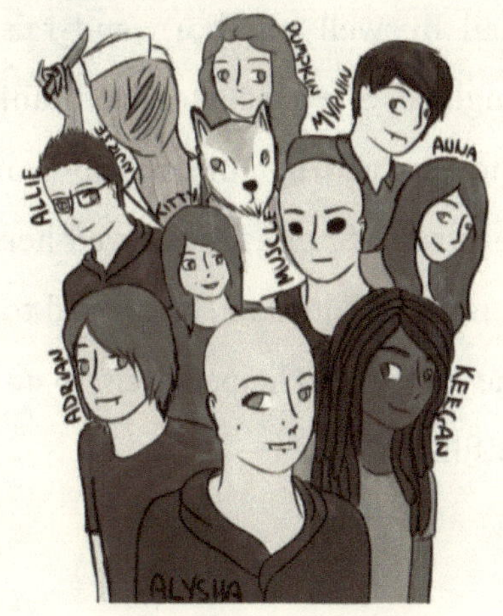

abuse, Adrianne became pregnant at age fifteen by an abusive man. She gave birth to her son at age sixteen in 2014, all on her own. She is now eighteen years old and after a five-year hiatus, is restarting school to gain her diploma.

*

GAIL BUSWELL
Gail was diagnosed with 13
personalities in 2002 at age 24

Gail Buswell was born and raised in a very small quiet village in England. She graduated from university with a degree in psychology, and pursued her dream job working with children on the autistic spectrum. She really enjoyed her job, as she is a deeply sensitive and compassionate soul. She loved to help others see the beautiful people they were, and helped them to unlock their potential to live happy and fulfilling lives.

*

KATT HART
Katt was diagnosed with hundreds
of personalities in 2011 at age 20
universe.systemx@gmail.com

Katt Hart was born in Yorkshire, England, but has since moved around a lot. She and her alters struggled in school and experienced a lot of bullying, which resulted in their having to drop out at age fifteen. They've attempted college several times, but have struggled to complete the courses, unfortunately. They are disabled, but draw as a way to earn small amounts of money and as a hobby. They spend a lot of time at home, and they cook and bake to keep themselves happy.

*

ROSEMARY HAWKINS
Rosemary was diagnosed with at
least 5 personalities in 2014 at age 46

Rosemary Hawkins was born in Queensland, Australia, to migrant parents. She is the middle child of five. Much of her childhood was spent caring for her siblings, as her mother suffered mental health issues and was often absent from family life. Rosemary's school years were spent at a strict Catholic convent school, an upbringing that would influence much of her formative years. She has married three times and has five children, four boys and a girl. Rosemary's interests lie in the area of mature age education and mental health education.

*

AMELIA JOUBERT
Amelia was diagnosed with 12
personalities in 2013 at age 15
Youtube.com/channel/UCW89GooAcoHK3922bN7Ve8g

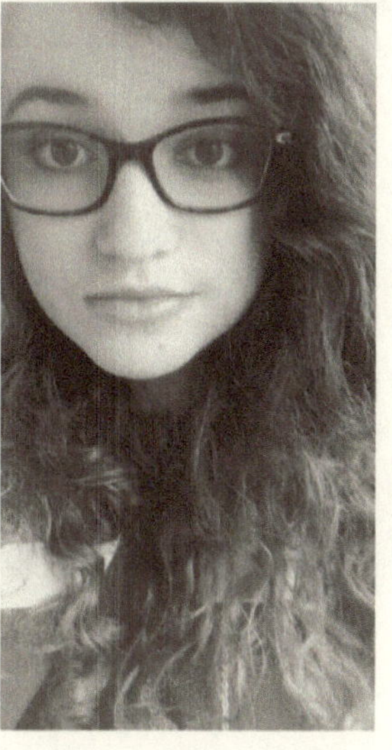

Amelia Joubert was born in Massachusetts and as a child moved to South Carolina, where she grew up and lives today. She is an avid reader and also enjoys writing. She has had several poems published, including in *Grief Diaries: Poetry & Prose and More.*

She is an animal lover and works pet sitting and babysitting. Amelia and her alter Scarlet are very active in the mental health community. They run an online support group for people with dissociative identity disorder, and a blog about their experiences. They also make YouTube videos about living with dissociative identity disorder. They are very passionate about helping others and educating people on mental health conditions.

*

AMANDA LINEBACK
Amanda was diagnosed with hundreds
of personalities in 2013 at age 31
themosaicofme@gmail.com

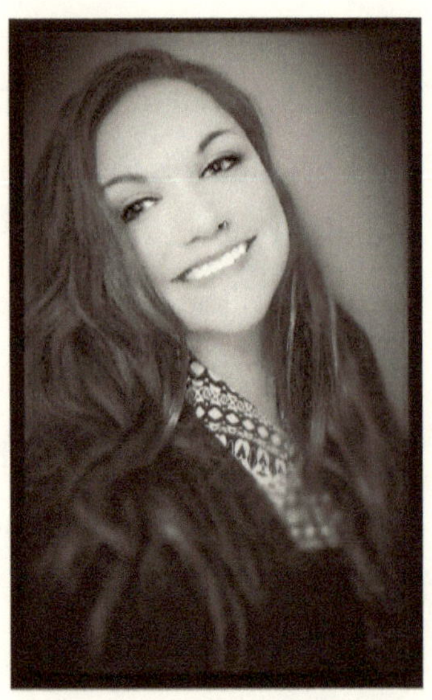

Amanda Lineback is a thirty-four-year-old mental health advocate from Evansville, Indiana. She graduated from F. J. Reitz High School in 2001. She is currently studying the metaphysical sciences, including energy healing, and Shamanism. She is in the beginning stages of starting a therapy group for people living with dissociative identity disorder.

Amanda currently lives in her hometown of Evansville, Indiana, with her two beautiful children, Jaylin and Jaden. She has a flair for art, and loves to draw and paint. She loves doing science experiments and art projects with her children. Amanda likes to be out in nature and in her free time can be found hunting for geodes, hiking, and geocaching.

*

JANE MACDONALD
Jane was diagnosed with 3 personalities in
2014 at age 35, and currently has 6 alters

Jane MacDonald was born and raised in the suburbs of a major Canadian city. She is the youngest of two children and grew up in a divorced home. She has college degrees in psychology and anthropology. She has lived with mental illness since a young age, but was only recently diagnosed with dissociative identity disorder. She is passionate about animals and is an advocate for individuals with mental health issues and those living in poverty.

*

CRYSTALIE MATULEWICZ
Crystalie was diagnosed with dissociative
identity disorder in 2015 at age 29
pafpac.org | lifewithouthurt.com | support@pafpac.org

Crystalie Matulewicz was born in northern New Jersey. She graduated with honors from Thomas Edison State University in 2015, earning her B.A. in psychology. Crystalie is currently pursuing her Master's in experimental psychology at the University of West Alabama. She has a special interest in affective

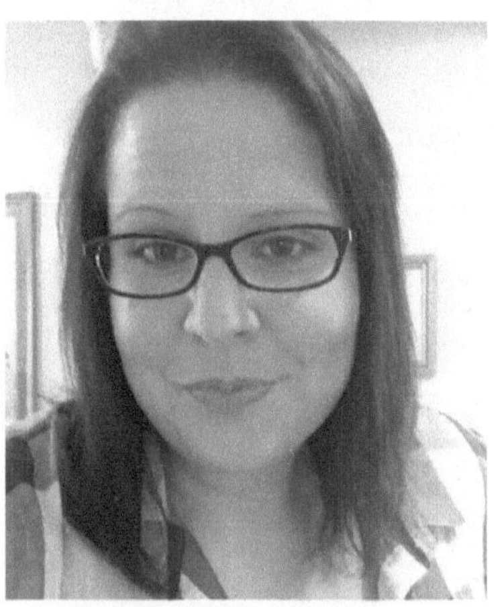

neuroscience and its applications in understanding sociopathy. In addition to working in retail, Crystalie is also the writer of the "Dissociative Living" blog at HealthyPlace, where she writes about DID from both educational and experiential points of view. She is also the author of "Life Without Hurt," her personal blog in which she writes about the escape from her family, her journey to freedom, and managing life with PTSD and DID (through a whole lot of therapy). Crystalie is the founder of PAFPAC, Promoting Awareness of Female Perpetrated Abuse of Children. She started the organization after completing her thesis on female-perpetrated abuse in 2015, in which she uncovered a significant lack of acknowledgment and support for victims. PAFPAC offers support for both male and female survivors of female-perpetrated abuse through its online support groups. Crystalie hopes to one day grow her organization and educate others on the reality of female-perpetrated child abuse.

*

ALICIA PETTIS
Alicia was diagnosed with 40
personalities in 2015 at age 16
goodbyeagony5145@gmail.com

Alicia Pettis was born in Scottsbluff, Nebraska. She lived there until moving to Hastings, Nebraska, at age eleven. Alicia struggled with school and peers, while also struggling to keep herself present. Even though she was fighting to do good in school, she always thought of others first. Her kindness spread to everyone, even if she didn't know them. She aspires to be a mental health therapist so she can help kids who are like her. She wants everyone to be happy and full of life, even if it means she has to be the person who pushes them to get to a better place.

*

SUNSHINE PURCELL
Denise was diagnosed with 17
personalities in 1995 at age 30
hello@sisterdiarieswithsunshine.com
www.sisterdiarieswithsunshine.com

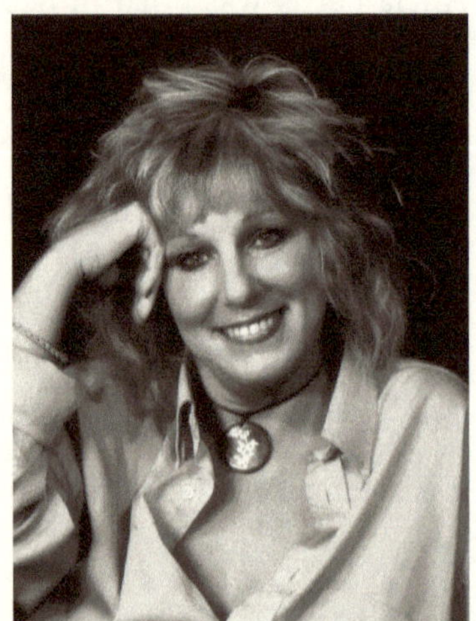

Denise Purcell was born the oldest of seven in Syracuse, New York. She is the mother of five girls and is a talented artist, published poet, and mental health advocate dedicated to bringing about better understanding and awareness of DID and other mental illnesses.

Sunshine and Andre, another alter, are gifted artists who authored Color Your Soul Whole, an adult coloring book. A prolific writer, her work has been published in numerous Grief Diaries titles. Sunshine has her own YouTube series, Sister Diaries with Sunshine, to raise awareness about living with DID. Learn more at www.sisterdiarieswithsunshine.com.

*

ERICKA REEVE
Ericka was diagnosed with over 25
personalities in 2013 at age 26
www.theweinme.com

Ericka Reeve was born in Chicago, Illinois, and has worked in the arts community her entire life. She is a writer, photographer, and model, and has published and sold her work since high school. Due to physical limitations, she is currently focused on writing and painting, though photography has always been her first love. She lives in the Midwest with her husband and their ferrets. Animals have always been a big part of her life, and that aspect of her has never left, even into adulthood.

Ericka has found amazing support through the online mental health community, and is now actively working to end the stigma surrounding mental health. DID is widely misunderstood and that nearly cost Ericka her life several times. Her and her parts are working within the community to end this damaging stigma, and to help those like herself.

*

CHRIS ROBIN
Chris was diagnosed with at least
7 personalities in 2013 at age 49

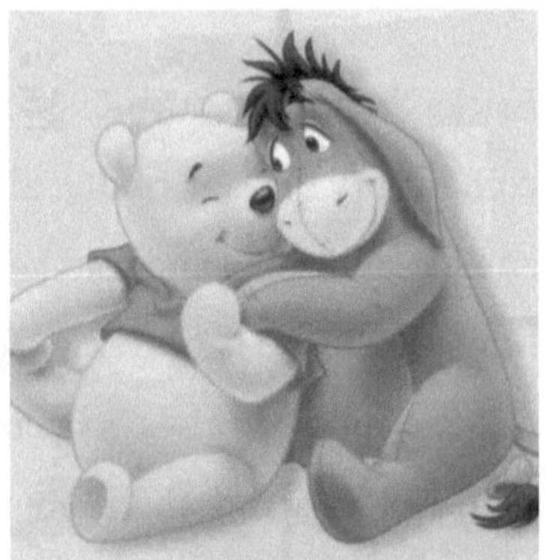

Chris Robin was born and raised in San Antonio, Texas. She went to Catholic school from third grade through high school. She earned her bachelor's degree in education from Our Lady of the Lake University in 1987, and began working as a teacher in San Antonio. She retired after thirty years of teaching first through fifth grade. She became a teacher and child advocate, and is now a local leader in her professional organization. She is a widower, a daughter, a lesbian, a teacher, a unionist, a sister, and a friend.

*

QUINN ROSE
Quinn was diagnosed with 9
personalities in 2016 at age 21

Quinn Rose was born in Alabama. Her parents loved her very much and she had a decent childhood. She grew up as a Christian. She was always a fun child but her parents feared that her fun side would get in the way of her future. She could make friends easily with anyone. She always made everyone feel so wonderful inside. She was definitely a little sunshine.

*

AYA SAKURA
Aya has been living with 7
personalities since childhood
aya-sakura@mail.com

Aya Sakura was born in 1997 in the Netherlands, and finished high school in 2014. Aya currently is a second-year student in human resource management and hopes to become a human resource professional. Her current goal is to find balance within her system and to improve communication.

*

MATTHEW SANCHEZ
Matthew was diagnosed with 8
personalities in 2015 at age 16

Matthew Sanchez was born in Minnesota in 1999.

*

FLOSS SCOTT
Floss was diagnosed with at least
4 personalities in 2016 at age 48

Floss Scott is the mother of three gorgeous, well-mannered adult children and three grandchildren, and is very proud of them all and loves them all to bits. Floss lost her first baby midway through the pregnancy, and it gutted her world. Everyone described her as a very strong, loving and caring person who could cope with anything, but her marriage broke down and she entered and ended various relationships, especially when they became very close to her. Floss has been a full-time working single mother since her youngest child was five. She put her life and soul into being a good mother and making sure her kids never went without. She enjoyed going out dancing, as this would be the only time she could go into her world of heaven without stress, sorrows, or storms; just the music and her. She also loves doing a variety of things including sewing and crafts, and always seems to do a good job though she doesn't know how or why. That's the mystery in her life.

*

PAULA SUNDWALL
Paula was diagnosed with dissociative amnesia in 2006 at age
36 and diagnosed with at least 4 personalities in 2014 at age 44

Paula Sundwall is forty-five years old and has raised two wonderful boys who are now eighteen and twenty-one. She is happily divorced and renting a room in a house with some friends. She lost her career and has had financial difficulties as well as work problems for the past five years because of her condition.

*
KERRYJANE VOTH
Kerryjane was diagnosed with
35 alters in 2013 at age 53
reverbnation.com/kerryjanevoth
reverbnation.com/corkandkerry
kerryjanevoth@gmail.com

Kerryjane Voth was born in Galt, Ontario, Canada (now known as Cambridge), in 1960. She is the second oldest of five children born to a fundamentalist Pentecostal ordained minister. After graduating grade twelve, Kerryjane attended several educational institutions including Guelph University, the University of Western Ontario, and Brock University where she studied journalism, science and visual arts. She is a graduate of Niagara College of Applied Arts & Technologies with a diploma in Business Administration and Human Resources.

She is an accomplished professional musician, singer and songwriter, and has been nominated for several music awards including the London Music Awards and the Jack Richardson Music Awards. She won a London Music Award in 2013 with her Celtic band, Cork&Kerry. In 2014, she won an Aeolian School of Music Scholarship Award. She has been studying voice and piano with the Aeolian School of Music since 2012.

Kerryjane is a mother of three and grandmother of seven. She lives in London, Ontario, with her service dog, Dax, and enjoys among other things spending time with her grandchildren and close friends, riding her bike and hiking.

FROM LYNDA CHELDELIN FELL

Thank you

I am deeply indebted to the writers of *Real Life Diaries: Through the Eyes of DID*. It requires tremendous courage to bare such vulnerability about a topic so misunderstood. The collective dedication to seeing this book published is a legacy to be proud of.

I'm especially grateful to my dear friend and coauthor Sunshine Purcell as well as Amelia Joubert. I admire both ladies immensely for their hard work to raise awareness and bring this book project to fruition. With such little clinical information available about DID, it is my sincere hope that readers who share the same path will find compassion and hope, family and friends will gain better understanding, and professionals will appreciate the candid and nonclinical insight narrated by writers across the globe.

Helen Keller once said, "Walking with a friend in the dark is better than walking alone in the light." By sharing our struggles, we learn that we aren't truly alone as we travel our journey, for there are others ahead of us, behind us, and right beside us. That is what Real Life Diaries is all about.

Lynda Cheldelin Fell

I
BY SUNSHINE

I have many friends, yet I've never met them;

I have many memories yet I can't remember.

I have a future but my past is my present;

if you were to ask who I am, it depends on the hour, day, minute.

I can draw and write poetry but I have no ability to do such

I can read but what have I read?

I can drive, but where did I go?

I can talk but the voice is unfamiliar.

I can touch but I have no sensation.

I have a heart, but I cannot feel.

I have a spirit, but it's been long broken.

I have a soul, but it is bound.

I've been a lot of places, but don't know where I've been.

I have many clothes, there are many sizes.

I have a house, but not a home.

I have a family, they are strangers.

I have goals, I can't achieve them.

I have dreams, they are nightmares.

I have thoughts, they are voices.

I am my own person, we are many.

I look into the mirror, there is no reflection.

I have emotions, they have names.

My eyes are green, they cannot see.

I am lonely, they are always with me.

I am me, I am them.

We are one person,

I   a m   m a n y .

ABOUT

Lynda Cheldelin Fell

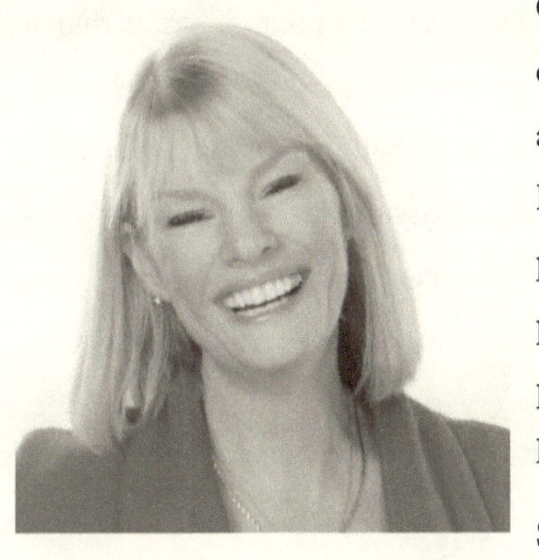

Considered a pioneer in the field of inspirational hope in the aftermath of hardship and loss, Lynda Cheldelin Fell has a passion for storytelling and producing groundbreaking projects that create a legacy of help, healing, and hope.

She is an international bestselling author and creator of the award-winning book series Grief Diaries and Real Life Diaries. Her repertoire of interviews include Dr. Martin Luther King's daughter, Trayvon Martin's mother, sisters of the late Nicole Brown Simpson, Pastor Todd Burpo of Heaven Is For Real, CNN commentator Dr. Ken Druck, and other societal newsmakers on finding healing and hope in the aftermath of life's harshest challenges.

Lynda's own story began in 2007, when she had an alarming dream about her young teenage daughter, Aly. In the dream, Aly was a backseat passenger in a car that veered off the road and landed in a lake. Aly sank with the car, leaving behind an open book floating face down on the water. Two years later, Lynda's dream became reality when her daughter was killed as a backseat passenger in a car accident while coming home from a swim meet. Overcome with grief, Lynda's forty-six-year-old husband suffered a major stroke that left him with severe disabilities, changing the family dynamics once again.

The following year, Lynda was invited to share her remarkable story about finding hope after loss, and she accepted. That cathartic experience inspired her to create groundbreaking projects spanning national events, radio, film and books to help others who share the same journey feel less alone. Now a passionate curator of stories, Lynda is dedicated to helping ordinary people share their own extraordinary journeys that touch the hearts of both reader and writer.

lynda@lyndafell.com | www.lyndafell.com

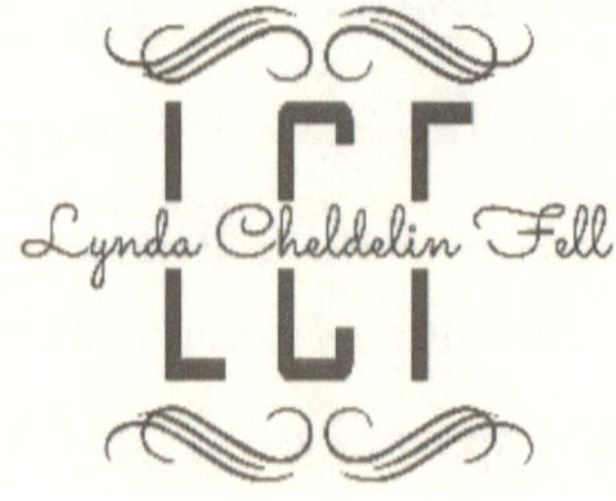

ALYBLUE MEDIA TITLES

Real Life Diaries: Living with Mental Illness

Real Life Diaries: Living with Endometriosis

Real Life Diaries: Living with Rheumatic Disease

Real Life Diaries: Living with a Brain Injury

Real Life Diaries: Through the Eyes of DID

Real Life Diaries: Through the Eyes of an Eating Disorder

Grief Diaries: Surviving Loss of a Spouse

Grief Diaries: Surviving Loss of a Child

Grief Diaries: Surviving Loss of a Sibling

Grief Diaries: Surviving Loss of a Parent

Grief Diaries: Surviving Loss of an Infant

Grief Diaries: Surviving Loss of a Loved One

Grief Diaries: Surviving Loss by Suicide

Grief Diaries: Surviving Loss of Health

Grief Diaries: How to Help the Newly Bereaved

Grief Diaries: Loss by Impaired Driving

Grief Diaries: Loss by Homicide

Grief Diaries: Loss of a Pregnancy

Grief Diaries: Hello from Heaven

Grief Diaries: Grieving for the Living

Grief Diaries: Shattered

Grief Diaries: Project Cold Case

Grief Diaries: Poetry & Prose and More

Grief Diaries: Through the Eyes of Men

Grief Diaries: Will We Survive?

Grief Diaries: Hit by Impaired Driver

Grammy Visits From Heaven

Grandpa Visits From Heaven

Faith, Grief & Pass the Chocolate Pudding

Heaven Talks to Children

God's Gift of Love: After Death Communication

Color My Soul Whole

Grief Reiki

Humanity's legacy of stories and storytelling
is the most precious we have.

DORIS LESSING

*

To share your story, visit
www.griefdiaries.com
www.RealLifeDiaries.com

PUBLISHED BY ALYBLUE MEDIA
Inside every human is a story worth sharing.
www.AlyBlueMedia.com

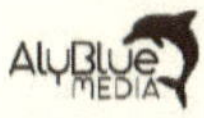

Shared joy is doubled joy;
shared sorrow is half a sorrow.
SWEDISH PROVERB

*